HOPE Rising

High Praise for
HOPE Rising

"Countless of our veterans returning from armed struggles overseas have experienced severe injuries; physical, emotional and psychological. For many, their return begins a long downward spiral of despair and a loss of hope. Some turn to drugs and alcohol for release. For far too many, suicide is the only relief. Casey Gwinn and Chan Hellman argue that returning hope to the lives of those who have served our nation should be our goal. I stand with them and endorse the message of this seminal book."

—Lt. General Jack Klimp (Ret.), United States Marine Corps

"*Hope Rising* will be an important source of help to those seeking to find ways to reduce the impact of adverse childhood experiences in order to live thriving, hope-filled lives. Dr. Chan Hellman and Casey Gwinn are the first researchers and authors to connect higher Hope Scores with reducing the impact of violence, trauma, and abuse. The potential benefit of implementing the science of hope throughout society is enormous if we truly want to meet the needs of the currently unrecognized multitudes of trauma-exposed adults and children."

— **Dr. Vincent J. Felitti,** Coauthor of the
Adverse Childhood Experiences (ACE) Study

"*Hope Rising* has a powerful message for anyone who has struggled with finding motivation to pursue their goals and dreams in life. So many great and successful people have found their success in high levels of hope and others have lost their way in the absence of hope. Casey Gwinn and Chan Hellman have given us a pathway to center our lives around hope and strategies to increase our own hope so we can be the fathers and men that we are called to be. Every reader will find inspiration, encouragement and radical hope within these pages."

— **Ted Bunch,** Co-Founder, A CALL TO MEN

"I have seen the miracle of hope in my oncology practice over and over again. Hope prolongs life. Casey Gwinn and Chan Hellman have written a book that translates the complex research into understandable concepts accessible to everyone. Cancer treatment has come so far and we are making more progress every day, but patients who choose hope will always be part of our success."

— **Dr. Marin Xavier,** Scripps Mercy Hospital, Cancer Center

"*Hope Rising* is a tremendous contribution to the national discussion about how to help survivors of violence, trauma, and abuse overcome the potentially devastating impacts that have such profound lifelong consequences. Casey Gwinn and Chan Hellman have made a powerful argument that the science of hope can help everyone to navigate trauma, abuse, and even the day to day adversities of life."

> — **Jacquelyn Campbell, Ph.D., R.N., FAAN,** Johns Hopkins University, School of Nursing

"*Hope Rising* is not just a book about the power of hope, it is a compassionate and scientific roadmap for building resilience and healing. If you're looking for an uplifting "handbook" on finding hope, look no further!"

> — **Ken Druck, Ph.D.**, Author of *The Real Rules of Life:*
> *Balancing Life's Terms with Your Own* and
> *Courageous Aging: Your Best Years Ever Reimagined*

"*Hope Rising* is a great book! Written in an engaging style, it should be a must-read for judges, attorneys, and others in the criminal and civil justice systems of this country. It changes our understanding of the essential role of hope in our justice system goals. If we focus on increasing the level of hope in the life of every trauma-exposed child in this country, we can save tens of millions of taxpayer dollars now spent on incarceration and correction. Those dollars can be re-purposed toward addressing the real needs of those living their lives with the toxic combination of rage and despair. *Hope Rising* provides the road map that gets us there."

> — **The Honorable Ronald B. Adrine**, Presiding Judge,
> Cleveland Municipal Court (Ret.)

"Casey Gwinn and Chan Hellman have done a superb job of revealing the transformative power of hope that resides within trauma, violence, and abuse. Though we all know on some level that hope is vital to our lives, they have given us the science to affirm our beliefs. In the process, they give us all a roadmap toward different, and better, lives."

> — **Gavin de Becker,** *New York Times* Best Selling Author of
> *The Gift of Fear: Survival Signals That Protect Us from Violence*

"*Hope Rising* is the most practical book imaginable on the power of hope. Casey Gwinn's experience as a prosecutor and storyteller and Chan Hellman's research expertise have combined to create a great book. They break down years of research into concepts that we can all apply to our lives whether our adversity comes from childhood or adulthood. We all need the reminder that hope is real and attainable no matter what we have experienced in life. I strongly recommend it to anyone who wants to feel the power of rising hope in their lives."

— **The Honorable Nancy O'Malley**, Alameda County District Attorney

"*Hope Rising* is a must read for anyone interested in happiness, spirituality, or well-being. Our broken world needs the power of hope now more than ever. The trauma and adversity that we all experience is the great destroyer of our God-given ability to hope. Casey Gwinn and Chan Hellman give us the strategies to restore the power to make our dreams a reality."

—**Chaplain (Colonel) William "Bill" Green Jr.**, US Army

"*Hope Rising* is the kind of book that every elected official and policy maker in the country should read when thinking about how we should measure success in working with and funding programs for those in need. Having faced significant adversity in my own life, I truly understand the power of hope. And now that we know there is genuine science behind it, I have no doubt that it can be used to help reduce populations in prison and juvenile-justice facilities across this country."

—California State President Pro Tem **Toni Atkins**

"I have seen the hope and resilience in domestic violence survivors and *Hope Rising* will help us better understand the science of hope and how rising hope can change the lives of those who struggle with discouragement, heartbreak, trauma, or even just the challenges of everyday life for those survivors and others. Casey Gwinn and Chan Hellman make the complex research accessible and understandable to everyone that wants to learn how to apply the science and see the power of rising hope in their lives and the lives of those they love."

—**Ruth Glenn**, President & CEO,
National Coalition Against Domestic Violence

HOPE
Rising

How the
Science of **HOPE**
Can Change
Your Life

Casey Gwinn, J.D.
& Chan Hellman, Ph.D.

NEW YORK

LONDON • NASHVILLE • MELBOURNE • VANCOUVER

HOPE Rising
How the **Science** *of* **HOPE** *Can Change Your Life*

Published in New York, New York, by Morgan James Publishing. Morgan James is a trademark of Morgan James, LLC. www.MorganJamesPublishing.com

The Morgan James Speakers Group can bring authors to your live event. For more information or to book an event visit The Morgan James Speakers Group at www.TheMorganJamesSpeakersGroup.com.

Morgan James BOGO™

A **FREE** ebook edition is available for you or a friend with the purchase of this print book.

CLEARLY SIGN YOUR NAME ABOVE

Instructions to claim your free ebook edition:
1. Visit MorganJamesBOGO.com
2. Sign your name CLEARLY in the space above
3. Complete the form and submit a photo of this entire page
4. You or your friend can download the ebook to your preferred device

ISBN 978-1-68350-965-3 paperback
ISBN 978-1-68350-966-0 eBook
Library of Congress Control Number:
2018934762

Cover Design by:
Rachel Lopez
www.r2cdesign.com

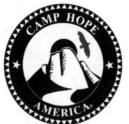

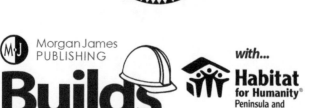

with...

Morgan James is a proud partner of Habitat for Humanity Peninsula and Greater Williamsburg. Partners in building since 2006.

Get involved today! Visit
MorganJamesPublishing.com/giving-back

To those who did not overcome, those who still long to thrive,
and to our children, and our children's children,
our hope for the future...

Table of Contents

A Note from the Authors

All the stories in this book are true. Hope is real. We have no need to make up any stories. Some names, personal characteristics and settings have been changed to protect the privacy of students, friends, family members, and acquaintances. Most of the names used are actual names and have been used with permission by the courageous and hope-centered young people and adults that want to release the shame and blame and publicly share their stories of hope rising.

Introduction

Lance

We were all gathered to take a group picture on the last night of camp at the first camping and mentoring program in America focused on children impacted by domestic violence. I (Casey) was on a ladder facing 60 children plus counselors and adult volunteers all lined up on the side of a hill for our group photo. A camper, a counselor, and our Program Coordinator, Maddie Orcutt, were missing. I did not know where they were. Determined to take the group photo, I focused my effort to get everyone to smile at the camera in my hand. Suddenly, every single head turned—looking past me out into a large, grassy field. I slowly turned to see Lance, a ten-year-old camper, running full speed across the field away from us. Maddie was sprinting behind him as Lance pulled away.

Lance was soaked in sweat running through camp and then down a dirt road away from camp. Pumping his arms, his face set in an angry grimace, oblivious to everyone and everything around him, he ran for nearly a mile. He ran for as long as he could. When he couldn't run any longer, he walked—a counselor, Jenny Dietzen, and Maddie trying to follow him.

I jumped in my Jeep and caught up with Lance, Jenny, and Maddie a little over a mile out of camp. As I drove alongside Lance, he refused to acknowledge my soft-spoken warnings that I would not let him run away from camp—that it was time to turn around and head back. Finally, I pulled ahead of Lance, blocked the road with my car, got out, and told Lance he could go no further. When he tried to push past me, I moved behind him and wrapped my arms around him in a restraint. As I took him to the ground, he tried to stab me with a shank hidden in the fold of his elbow. I removed the shank and held him in a bear hug. He swore, cursed, struggled, and raged at me.

Lance had been triggered from something said or done to him—something no one could later identify—when he ran away at about 7 PM. Hours earlier, he had said he was having the "greatest week of his life"—a week filled with laughter, adventure, and new friends. And yet, white-hot anger now compelled him down the dirt road as he struggled to deal with complex emotions on the last night of camp. I would later find out he had intended to "run" back to his group foster home in Stockton, CA, which is nearly 250 miles from Arroyo Grande, CA, so he could try to find his mother. She had lost her parental rights to him years earlier because of domestic violence and drug abuse.

As I held Lance on the side of the dirt road with the setting sun in the distance, sitting directly behind him on the ground, restraining him with his arms pinned to his sides, the ten-year-old boy continued to rage at me. He threatened to kill me, screaming epithets. I wanted to let him go but I feared for his safety and mine if he could get his hands and arms free. We were both wet with sweat as he struggled for his freedom and I resisted with every ounce of strength I had left. Nearby Maddie and Jenny sat quietly, turned away, not wanting to be witnesses to this terrible moment of intersection in our lives. Minutes passed. An hour went by...

My words were careful, thoughtful, and only loving. "I care too much about you to let you run away from camp, Lance." "You have a right to be angry." "I am so sorry for all the bad things people have done to you." "You did not deserve it, Lance." "You deserve to be loved." "You can get through this and have a great future." "Breathe with me, Lance." "Try to relax and think about the happiest part of your week." "I can't wait to see who you become." "You can be a man of kindness." "You can use your pain to help other kids someday, Lance." "You are a leader, Lance." "You can be a great role model for other kids someday." "Breathe with me, Lance." "Feel my heart beating and my chest moving up and down and try to follow me."

One hour and twenty minutes into the restraint protocol, I tried to engage Lance in a conversation about computers as his rage wore down and he slowly stopped fighting my arms wrapped around him as we sat on the side of the road. Another staff member, named Peggy, joined me on the side of the road. First, Peggy and I talked to each other, intentionally ignoring Lance. We talked about the camp slideshow that night. We talked about how much we liked computers and what a great slideshow we were going to have that night with all the kids if we had time to get it done. Then, we began to engage him. Peggy asked, "Do you have a computer, Lance?" Quietly, he said, "Yes. A Mac." I saw my opening. "Lance, I really need to finish the slideshow for the week so we can all see the entire week of camp tonight and celebrate together. The kids all really want to see the slideshow, but it is not done yet. If we're able to finish it, it will make everyone so happy. Will you help me with the slide show?"

He was fully present again. "Sure." Finally, a breakthrough. "Lance, if I let go of you, will you promise not to run away? Will you promise to get in my Jeep with me and go back to camp?" "I will," said Lance without the slightest trace of anger or resentment. "After you help me with the slideshow, you can choose from two options. I can get someone to drive you four hours back to Stockton tonight or you can wait until tomorrow and go home with the rest of the kids. It is your choice." Lance agreed to let me know his decision later. I let go of him, helped him up and we got in the car and drove back to camp. I quickly gave him my Mac and put him to work in the dining room editing pictures from the week for the slideshow. I sat next to him as he looked through the pictures. He paused, looked at me, and said, "Can I stay with you, just you, until it is time for me to make my decision?" Hope was rising in his life. He was finding a pathway forward. "Of course, Lance."

An hour later, 60 children poured into the dining room yelling, cheering, and ready for ice cream sundaes and the slideshow of the week. After they had all gathered, I publicly praised and thanked Lance for helping me with the slideshow. The entire room erupted in clapping for Lance and he smiled, stood, and waved to the crowd—not the slightest trace of the murderous rage he had directed toward me just 90 minutes earlier. The slideshow was a glorious 20 minutes of cheers and laughs as the kids saw themselves in pictures, set to music, of the entire week of Camp HOPE America at Lopez Lake. Lance stayed by my side the whole time. Minutes after the slideshow ended, Lance leaned close to me and said, "I have made my decision." "What are you going to do, Lance?", I asked. "I want to stay at camp tonight and go home tomorrow with everyone else." He paused. "And I have one other question." "What is it, Lance?" "Can I come back to camp next year?" "Of course, Lance. We all love you. And it will be great to have you back next year."

I want Lance to come back to camp next year and the year after that. I want Lance to find a way to hope and healing. Lance will never get any judgement or condemnation from me. No shame. No blame. No condemnation. Just the best chance we can give him to stay out of juvenile hall, jail, and prison—the best chance we can give him to never beat or rape a woman. We will do all we can to help him learn to get through his trauma, rage, and pain. Lance needs rising hope in his life. In fact, rising hope—measurable, rising hope—is his best chance to break the vicious generational cycle of violence that has claimed his mother, his father, and, most likely, other family members.

Five years ago, I didn't know hope was measurable. During twenty years as a prosecutor, I never learned that hope was a science. I didn't know hope changes the destiny of the trauma survivor, cardiac patient, paralyzed athlete, widow, abused child, cancer survivor, natural disaster victim, and battered woman. I didn't know what a Hope score was. I thought hope was a wish, a dream, a vague idea about a better future. What I have learned in the last five years has changed my life. I learned it from my co-author, Dr. Chan Hellman, one of the leading hope researchers in America.

In 2012, I was in Tulsa working with the Family Safety Center, a multi-agency collaborative where many agencies come together under one roof to help victims of family violence and their children. The director's name is Suzann Stewart and she was partnering with the Charles and Lynn Schusterman Family Foundation to improve the services of the Family Safety Center. She brought in the nonprofit I am honored to lead with our CEO Gael Strack, called Alliance for HOPE International, to help with their planning for the future. Suzann said she wanted me to meet Dr. Chan Hellman from the University of Oklahoma (OU) before I headed back home to San Diego later that day. She said Chan was a statistical psychologist researching "hope." It seemed immediately like a blind date opportunity with a bad ending. Who wants to be friends with a statistical psychologist? And you can't even measure hope anyway, can you?

I didn't know until years later that Chan felt the same way about getting together with me, an attorney from California. He wanted to be home swimming in his pool with his granddaughter. Who wants to be friends with a lawyer?

Suzann was relentless though and so we settled on a Skype call while Chan was enjoying his pool and I was in downtown Tulsa pretending to be interested in Chan's life as a statistical psychologist. Little did Chan and I know this meeting would change the trajectory of both of our personal and professional lives.

The first conversation was short. Chan tried to explain Dr. Rick Snyder's Theory of Hope and used words like "pathways," "willpower," and "waypower." He said hope was measurable. I didn't get it. I talked about Camp HOPE America and Family Justice Centers, places like the Tulsa Family Safety Center, where all the services for victims of abuse come together in one place. We had no published research, but I was sure our work was making a difference because of the anecdotal stories coming so often from the adults and children getting help and support. The brief talk, however, about "goals" and "pathways" got me thinking actively about Chan's assertion that hope was measurable. Could this be true? How would you verify it? How could you change someone's level of hope? Would higher levels of hope matter in someone's life?

Five years later, this meeting has led to the science of hope becoming a central philosophy of the Family Justice Center movement (www.familyjusticecenter.com), Camp HOPE America (www.camphopeamerica.com), and a host of other programs connected with Alliance for HOPE International (www.allianceforhope.com). Now, with Chan's Hope Research Center at OU leading the way, hope science is moving across the United States. A brief Skype call with two reluctant, old, introverted, childhood trauma survivors would change everything for each of us. We pray it changes things for many others too.

This book will teach you things about hope you have never heard or read anywhere else. It will challenge what you have believed about hope. It will change the way you talk about your life. It is not a long book, but it is backed up by hundreds of research studies (some of which are referenced at the end of this book) done in the last twenty years by a growing number of hope researchers. It is not just our opinion or personal belief treatise. It started out as a "theory" with a researcher and psychologist, Dr. C.R. ("Rick") Snyder at the University of Kansas twenty years ago. It moved further with the work of Dr. Shane J. Lopez, who studied under Rick Snyder and later became a Senior Research Scientist at Gallup.

The findings about hope are amazingly consistent from study to study and they have given us a message to deliver. Hope is not just an idea. Hope is not simply an emotion. It is far more than a feeling. It is not a wish or even an expectation. Hope is about goals, willpower, and pathways. A person with high hope has goals, the motivation to pursue them, and the determination to overcome obstacles and find pathways to achieve them.

Hope is a science with identifiable, measurable elements. It is measurable and it is malleable. You can give your level of hope (goals, willpower, and pathways) in life a "score" and measure it in others as well. Then, you can increase your Hope score by intentional strategies. Rising hope is predictive of short-term and long-term positive outcomes in people's lives. If you apply the science of hope to your life, it will change you. If you embrace the language of hope, you will talk differently, act more intentionally, and live your life with greater purpose than you ever have before.

Our personal goal should be to act in ways that increase our own Hope scores. Our relational goals should be to increase Hope scores in the lives of those we love. Our professional goals as employers should be to increase the Hope scores of our employees. Our goals in serving the poor, the homeless, the traumatized, combat veterans, the mentally ill, and the victimized should be to increase hope in their lives. If we are not increasing hope, what are we doing? What if we change our own hope levels and then start increasing hope in the lives of those we serve, work with, and love? What might the world look like?

Social service organizations, criminal and civil justice system agencies, medical facilities, educational institutions, places of worship, the military, and businesses across America need the message of hope described in this book. We should be measuring hope and then working to increase it. Once we increase our own hope, we can start to increase the hope of those around us. We should be creating it in government and non-government programs. Non-profit organizations getting funded from the local, state, or federal government should be measuring whether they are producing hope as an intended outcome. Philanthropists, private foundations, and donors should be investing in the organizations that can prove they are hopegivers.

We should be all about rising hope, but often we are not. Why? Many don't know about the science of hope. Many others aren't willing to work for it. We need to make the decision to learn about it and then we need to be willing to do the work to get higher hope in our lives.

With nearly 2,000 published studies, it is no longer just a theory. It must be called what it is—a science. Chan has now published a host of peer-reviewed studies on hope through his work at the University of Oklahoma and is involved in more than 75 other current hope studies. Hope is real.

Our careers and our work in writing this book have been heavily informed by the work of Dr. Rick Snyder and Dr. Shane Lopez from the University of Kansas. We will talk more about their work later. Books like *Ghosts from the Nursery* and *Scared Sick* by Robin Karr-Morse, talking about trauma and its relation to brain development, are important contributions to our research when we think about what damages hope in people's lives.

Dr. Vincent Felitti and Dr. Robert Anda and their *Adverse Childhood Experiences (ACE)* Study have changed our view of everything we do in this work. The ACE Study, first conducted by Anda and Felitti, is the most predictive study ever done on the impact of childhood trauma on adult illness, disease, victimization, and criminality. The ACE Index produces a score between 0-10 related to the trauma you suffered during childhood. The higher the score, the worse the long-term consequences are in your life without intervention. We will talk more about the ACE Study later in the book.

We also love *The Body Keeps the Score* by Bessel van der Kolk. Bessel van der Kolk has helped many better understand how bad things that happen to us can impact our emotional, spiritual, and physical health. *The Body Keeps the Score* was, and still is, one of the most helpful books ever written on how trauma in life affects short and long-term health. It has helped tens of thousands of people around the world to finally understand their mental health struggles, damaged organs, poor physical health, and so many other impacts from unmitigated trauma and toxic stress on the human body. The message was powerful: The body absorbs the impacts of things people experience in utero, as children, and throughout their lives—and the consequences on mental and physical health can be devastating.

But *The Body Keeps the Score* did not give people the answers on how to mitigate those impacts with rising hope. It did not provide a way to produce a counteracting, strength-based, positive "score" that a person can pursue to undo the profound, long-term consequences of unmitigated trauma and toxic stress on the body and the brain. If childhood trauma makes you more likely to be an alcoholic, what do you do about it? If sexual abuse makes you more likely to be obese or bulimic, what do you do about it? Everyone wants answers to changing the endings that are predicted from bad things that happen in our lives. Many strategies are helpful but the science of hope is central to these answers.

Brené Brown's work around shame, blame, and vulnerability in *Daring Greatly* and *Braving the Wilderness* has also played a role for us in helping us connect pain and hope. Pain can become power. Honesty and vulnerability play important roles in that journey. Brené loves to say you cannot give what you do not have. This is true with hope. You cannot give hope to others if you don't have hope. The science of hope can add more to these important concepts for each of us.

Nadine Burke Harris' book, *The Deepest Well: Healing the Long-Term Effects of Childhood Adversity*, is also an important resource in this conversation. Nadine comes from a medical perspective and shares her amazing work at the Center for Youth Wellness in San Francisco. The truth is though that most of the needs of children and adults will not be met in a hospital or medical facility. They will be met in the day to day of lives lived with an understanding of how trauma impacts us and strategies that release the trauma and increase hope in our lives.

Two years ago, I published *Cheering for the Children: Creating Pathways for Children Exposed to Trauma. Cheering for the Children* was one of the first books written to the general public to begin looking at how to alleviate the consequences of adverse childhood experiences. It looked at many things we have learned in our work with traumatized adults and children. But it did not go where this book goes. This book makes the case that rising hope—in fact, a higher Hope score—is the most powerful way to allay the effects of childhood trauma, toxic stress, and painful, difficult experiences throughout your life. Rising hope doesn't *eliminate* the impact of trauma, but it *mitigates* trauma. Hope helps to put trauma in the rearview mirror.

The sooner we get to rising hope the better. Children need rising hope as soon as possible after trauma. Those who lose a loved one need to know that hope can rise again. Those struggling with depression can improve their symptoms. After the loss of a job, a marriage, or a house, rising hope is crucial. And once we have greater hope, it can influence us, those we love, friends, neighbors, and co-workers and allow us to be hopegivers ourselves.

By the grace of God, Chan and I have both navigated through our own personal journeys with childhood adversity to pursue the power of hope. For the first time in this book, we have shared our honest, personal stories. Everyone has a story and very often pain, loss, and trauma from childhood relate to our struggles to be people with high levels of hope in our lives. The good news is we can all overcome the people and experiences that may have robbed us of hope and caused us great pain. In this book, we will ask you to reflect on your own life. It is only right that we are personally honest about our lives. Here are short pieces from each of our stories:

Chan

I grew up in a small farming community with a population under 1,000 and a graduating high school class of 21 students. We rented a small farmhouse when I was in the fourth grade having just moved back to NW Oklahoma from Tulsa. This was the end of the Vietnam War and my parents were flower children "hippies" who protested the war and engaged in the drug culture. My father became a drug dealer when I was in elementary school and had several hidden locations where he grew marijuana. My "job" was to help cultivate, harvest, and package the marijuana into ¼ to one ounce bags. My dad used to take me on drug sales that I now believe were his effort to reduce the chance of violence by buyers…

When I entered the seventh grade my parents got a loan to buy a small house in town. Moving from the rented farm, I now lived in a house that everyone would see. This "new" house had a leaky roof and a dirt floor basement that would flood in every rainstorm. At about this same time, I was being bullied and tormented by one of the children in my class who now lived on the same block. I not only lived in fear and shame due to the "family business" but also in fear for my day-to-day physical and emotional safety from a bully.

Within a few months of moving into our house, my parents announced they were going to divorce—throwing my world into further turmoil. My dad moved back to Tulsa with his girlfriend and had limited interaction with us. Of course, child support was non-existent. I believe my mother tried her best, but spent a brief time hospitalized for depression. She had dropped out of high school, and was eventually able to get a job in the city 40 miles away. Perhaps the pressure was too much, as she just stopped coming home…

Casey

I don't remember the first time I was afraid of my dad. It was early in my life. He would get angry and frustrated and it was always my fault if he was mad. He wasn't always mad though. He was kind and loving too. Maybe that's why it was confusing. I remember sometimes being happy when he was mad at my sisters or my brother. It wasn't me. And when he was nice it was the best.

My dad was all-powerful. He seemed to never make a mistake and I learned early not to question him or try to talk to him when he was mad. Many years later a therapist would ask me why I never told my dad how his anger and violence made me feel when I was a child. I got up and walked out of her office. I had to find a better therapist.

Dad didn't call it violence. He called it discipline. "Spare the rod and spoil the child." "Quit your crying or I will give you something to cry about." It always seemed like a stupid statement since I had something to cry about—that is why I was crying. But I learned not to cry. I learned not to show an ounce of emotion when he whipped me. The only emotion I remember was anger. I looked forward to when he calmed down and told me that it hurt him more than it hurt me, even though I thought that was horseshit. But I never would have said horseshit in my Dad's presence.

I remember many instances when my father held me down while my mom rubbed a bar of soap in my mouth and across my teeth and then made me swallow. I never said a swear word but there was clearly something I had said that was an unforgiveable sin. For the life of me, I cannot remember one thing I said that ever deserved the bar of soap in my mouth that made me gag and feel like I was choking.

He did to me what his father had done to him but not as bad. After my dad died in 2009, I learned that he was punched in the head by his father every day to be awakened when he was a child. "Wee Willie Wee, wake up," my grandfather would say before his fist greeted my dad's head. When my mom told me in 2010, she wondered out loud, "It is amazing your father was as normal as he was given all those times he got hit in the head as a child." I asked her how it stopped. She said when my dad was 13 he woke up one day before my grandfather came in the room and as my grandfather approached him my dad, now 6'0 tall, stood up to my grandfather, balled his fists and said, "If you ever hit me again, I will kill you." Then, my mom said matter of factly, "And you know…his father never hit him again." But I believe the damage was done…

You will find the rest of my journey in Chapter 18. You will find the rest of Chan's personal account of his life in Chapter 19. You will also see other stories of triumph over trauma and adversity from many others. Some wanted to write their own story in the first person. Others asked us to tell their story for them.

We have written this book together. You will only see "I" in a few stories at the beginning of chapters. The rest of the time you will see us write as "we" or sometimes in the third person when describing one of our personal experiences. This book is very much about what "we" have learned together in our lives about the power of hope.

Hope is measurable, malleable, and attainable. It is not wishful thinking. It can drive our personal and our professional lives once we understand it and apply the science to our lives and our organizations. Lance needs it. I need it. Chan needs it. You need it.

Hope Rising: How the Science of Hope Can Change Your Life is the third book ever written for the public on the science of hope. Rick Snyder and Shane Lopez wrote the first two. They have both passed away. Rick died of cancer. Shane died after a two-year battle with depression. Rick and Shane inspired us to be more honest about our own lives and dig deeper into the life-saving power of hope. Come along; join us. You will never be the same again. You will make different choices. You will set different goals for your life. You will use different words and language. You will find power you never imagined possible if you are willing to do the work. Once you achieve high hope, you will be able to help others achieve it as well. Hope is measureable. Hope is malleable. Hope changes the world. Spread the word.

Casey Gwinn, J.D.

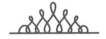

Chapter 1

A Culture of Hope

"Hope is the bridge between the impossible and the possible."
—Joseph Bellezzo, M.D.

Diane

On Thursday, November 30, 2017, Diane McGrogan was having chest pain. She was on her way to get her nails done for her company Christmas party on Saturday night. She called her sister, Joanne, and told her about the pain but said she would just pull over and wait until it passed. Joanne told her to drive straight to the hospital and she would meet her there. Diane argued but eventually turned around and headed to Sharp Memorial Hospital in San Diego. On her way, she called her boyfriend, Ron, and he said he would meet her at the hospital too. At the hospital, she parked her car and walked herself toward the ER. As she approached the automatic doors, the pain was blinding. She started to feel light-headed. The door got blurry. She sat down on a bench right outside the door of the ER. The pain shot down her right leg. She couldn't make either leg move. Everything started going dark. Diane fell fast and hard off the bench.

A nurse named Jessica rushed out to Diane, found no heartbeat, and began cardiopulmonary resuscitation (CPR). They attempted manual CPR as they brought her lifeless body into the ER on a gurney. Doctors, nurses, and technicians formed a team and worked to save her. Despite CPR, cardiac defibrillation, and medicine, Diane did not regain circulation. They soon hooked her up to a Lucas CPR machine, an automated chest compression device. The Lucas CPR provides consistent lifesaving, uninterrupted chest compressions to reduce the chances of neurological damage in patients who suffer sudden cardiac arrest.

Dr. Joseph Bellezzo, the Chief of Emergency Medicine at Sharp Memorial Hospital, was on duty that day. He saw the frantic team of doctors and nurses at work on her. In the life and death moments of the team checking vital signs, performing compressions to her chest, installing the Lucas CPR device, and yelling commands back and forth, Bellezzo determined that Diane's heart was not capable of sustaining life in that moment. An EKG confirmed it, Diane had suffered a massive heart attack. The coronary cath-lab team was activated, but it would be 20 minutes before they would be ready for her. Bellezzo made the split-second decision to use a new procedure he had been perfecting (in conjunction with his colleague Dr. Zack Shinar)—the use of a heart-lung bypass machine—to try to save the life of patients in cardiac arrest who would otherwise die in the ER. During the chaos of CPR, in a matter of minutes, Bellezzo made incisions in Diane's femoral artery and vein—not in an operating room but in the Emergency Department. He next inserted wires into the blood vessels to clear a pathway to her heart, and then "cannulated" her (inserted tubes). Cannulation allows blood to be drawn away from the failing heart, passing it through a machine that provides needed oxygen to the blood, and returns the freshly oxygenated blood back to the body—effectively providing total heart-lung bypass. The procedure, called extracorporeal membrane oxygenation (ECMO), kept her alive. It was a complete bypass of both her stopped heart and lungs. The procedure, performed in a matter of minutes, is life-support for the dead.

They would later find Diane had 95% blockage of her left anterior descending (LAD) artery. Considered the most important of three main coronary arteries to the heart, the LAD supplies over half of the heart muscle with blood. When the left anterior descending artery is blocked, right at the beginning of the vessel, it is known as the "widowmaker" because most die without immediate medical intervention. The "widowmaker" caused Diane's heart to suddenly stop beating and prevented the medical team from getting it started again. Diane, with 95% occlusion to her LAD, would have died on November 30, 2017 without ECMO and the life-giving team of highly skilled doctors, nurses, and technicians. Once on ECMO, Diane was rushed into surgery that first night to clear the blockage, insert a stent (scaffolding to keep the blood vessel open), and get her heart pumping again on its own.

I (Casey) found out Friday morning that my friend, Diane, was in critical condition from a massive heart attack. I talked to her sister, Joanne, and her boyfriend, Ron, and then felt compelled to head straight to the hospital to support both of them as best I could. When I arrived at Sharp, Joanne was just getting there after a few hours of sleep at home. I did not know Joanne well but I knew in my heart that I needed to be there for her. Ron arrived a couple hours later and we settled into the waiting room. Sitting in a hospital Intensive Care Unit waiting room, wondering if the news will be good or bad, is a terrible place to find hope. The unknown, the shock, and the fear are all overwhelming. As I was sitting with Joanne and Ron, Dr. Joe Bellezzo walked into the waiting room. He was kind, patient, and thoughtful. He explained that Diane was alive but that there were no guarantees. She had experienced manual and mechanical CPR for 32 minutes before they put her on heart-lung bypass. There was no way to know yet if she had suffered brain damage. There was a risk of clots, stroke, and infections. There was no way of knowing how long it might be before they could try to remove her tracheotomy, take her off the machine, and see if her heart could sustain life. It could be days or even weeks.

Joe Bellezzo had met Ron and Joanne the night before but he asked who I was. I told him I was the former City Attorney of San Diego and that Diane and I used to work together. He asked what I was doing now and I told him of my work with Alliance for HOPE International. He said he believed in the power of hope and thought Diane had a great chance of surviving. The timing was amazing. I was sitting and talking to a doctor who believed in hope at the same time that Chan and I were writing a book about the science of hope. I told him briefly about our book and Joe Bellezzo said, "We need to talk more. I always say that hope is the bridge between the impossible and the possible. When I say it around some of my doctor friends, they all get a good laugh." I knew one of the reasons I was supposed to be at the Sharp Hospital. Joe Bellezzo had some things to teach me about hope.

It would be four days on ECMO before her heart was able to recover and function without mechanical assistance. Every day was filled with ongoing 24-hour support. A small, elite group of highly trained nurses manage the ECMO program at Sharp Memorial Hospital and are trained to monitor and care for these type of heart-lung bypass patients.

Total heart-lung bypass in this circumstance is called veno-arterial extracorporeal membrane oxygenation (VA-ECMO). In adults, VA-ECMO is most often used to support open heart surgery patients who need prolonged cardiac support. It is also commonly used as life-support in newborns born prematurely, or with serious birth defects, that require vital organ support. When ECMO was first developed and machines were created in the

1980s, no one ever imagined that they would be used to resuscitate Emergency Department patients suffering massive cardiac arrest. But as Dr. Ian Malcolm said in Jurassic Park, "Life…finds a way."

On July 28, 2010, Drs. Bellezzo and Shinar were the first Emergency Physicians in the country to successfully use VA-ECMO in the Emergency Department (ED)—when they saved a cardiac patient named Ralph who suffered a widowmaker. Bellezzo and his team have now used ED ECMO to save many patients who would have otherwise died from massive cardiac arrest. Sharp has become one of the leading VA-ECMO hospitals in the United States. Bellezzo and Shinar, along with Dr. Scott Weingart, now travel the world training other doctors in the procedure—helping them to save more and more patients who suffer refractory cardiac arrest—most of whom would have otherwise died. They call themselves "resuscitationists." The high hope they carry in their work is saving lives.

But none of this is the best part of the story.

In 2008, using traditional resuscitation techniques, the survival rate at Sharp Memorial Hospital for out-of-hospital cardiac arrest patients was 8%—in line with national averages. By 2014, four years after implementing VA-ECMO for refractory cardiac arrest, the survival rate jumped to a stunning 28%. One could easily attribute the improved survival to the use of the life-saving procedure. But even after adjusting for the VA-ECMO cases, the survival rate for cardiac arrest patients not receiving VA-ECMO was still 28%! How could this be? Why had the survival rates for all major cardiac event patients in the ER risen so dramatically in just four years?

Dr. Bellezzo, after evaluating every variable, concluded that his doctors and nurses had changed their views of the potential for survival. "In 2008, there was a nihilism in our ER. Most of those coming into the ER with cardiac arrest were going to die. There was nothing we felt we could do about it. 8% survival means 92% failure—and that is awfully depressing. But the VA-ECMO procedure began to change that. Our teams started seeing that we could save far more people than they first believed and the power of hope became a core value. Hope became the bridge between the impossible and the possible. Once our doctors and nurses believed they could save more patients, our survival rates went up regardless of whether the cardiac patient received VA-ECMO or not. We created a culture of hope. Doctors and nurses believed we could save more people and then patients and their families began to believe."

The culture of hope is now saving more lives than ever at Sharp Memorial Hospital. In fact, Drs. Bellezzo, Shinar, and Weingart, are inspiring Emergency Department (ED) physicians around the globe. They host an international educational podcast to educate doctors called the ED ECMO Podcast (www.edecmo.org). And they host an international ED ECMO Conference called Reanimate (www.reanimateconference. com)—teaching resuscitationists all over the world to embrace their growing culture of hope.

Bellezzo's dream is now to put a mechanical chest compression device on every ambulance with hopes to identify and transport patients with cardiac arrest. Bellezzo says it best, "We can save many who are truly too vital to die." Some have even proposed ECMO implementation in the pre-hospital setting. In France, where the transport of cardiac arrest patients is logistically challenging, pre-hospital ECMO is gaining support. In one case, ECMO was used to save a patient who had a major heart attack on the floor of the Louvre in Paris—amid art patrons and famous paintings dating back hundreds of years.

Sometimes hope is dramatic like Diane's harrowing and life-saving journey through an Emergency Department in San Diego after a heart attack. Sometimes it is found in the physical restraint of a rage-filled boy on a dirt road by someone who loves him enough to keep him from hurting himself like Casey did with Lance. And sometimes you can see it in the quiet activities of everyday life. Martin Luther said, "Everything that is done in the world is done by hope." What made the difference for Diane? A culture of hope.

Once we understand hope, we can choose to believe in it and then work for it. After we do it individually, we can recruit others to join us. This allows us to create a culture of hope with others that has even greater power than individual hope. We will talk later about the research around collective hope—the power of a group of people who all have rising hope.

Diane is alive today because of the culture of hope that has been established in the Emergency Department at Sharp Memorial Hospital. An amazing team believed they could save her...then her boyfriend, Ron...and her sister, Joanne, believed. Then, her friends and family believed. In Joanne's words, "The grace of God and the power of hope saved my sister." In Ron's view, as an engineer, "The science of ECMO opened the door to the science of hope." It is a sacred honor to love someone who has been touched by death. Ron and Joanne will cherish that honor for many years to come with Diane.

The most recent research on VA-ECMO is now finding "save rates" as high as 40% in Minnesota as doctors perfect the procedure and implement Dr. Bellezzo's protocols faster and faster in cardiac arrest patients. The notion of "ED-ECMO" is becoming a philosophy never imagined before 2011 and it is beginning to save lives in other emergency departments all around the world. So far, just 13 hospitals in the country have implemented ED-ECMO but many more will learn what it means to have a culture of hope in the years ahead.

We believe every company should consider what a culture of hope might look like. This is not just a concept for the medical community. How would it change the legal profession? What if every element of the criminal and civil justice system including the courts of this country focused on hope? What about banking, manufacturing, the service industry, or the military? What would a hope-centered law enforcement agency look like? What about mental health facilities, senior living centers, and nursing homes? Could every elementary, middle, and high school create a culture of hope? What if every technical school, community college, and university operated with hope as a central tenet?

What if we all lived in a culture of hope? What if we all worked in a culture of hope? What if everyone dealing with challenges and difficulties found a place where hope was so high that it invaded their lives as they soon as they arrived? What if returning combat veterans immediately found higher hope? What if our families had a culture of hope? What if companies had a culture of hope? What if our relationships had high hope? What if every marriage had high hope?

We share Joe Bellezzo's view. Hope is real. Hope is the bridge between the impossible and the possible. We need many more bridge builders in this country.

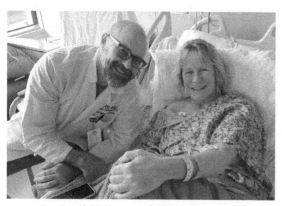

Dr. Joseph Bellezzo with Diane McGrogan

Joe Bellezzo says his colleagues and friends laugh when he says hope is real and when he talks about hope being the "bridge between the impossible and the possible." They find it hard to believe it could be a science or any part of "real" medicine. Diane McGrogan is certain they are wrong. Twelve days after suffering her heart attack she met with the Emergency Department team at Sharp Memorial Hospital that saved her life and thanked her hopegivers. They were real people with high hope—doctors and nurses and technicians who work in a culture of hope.

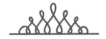

Chapter 2

What is Hope?

"Hope is a good thing, maybe the best of things, and no good thing ever dies."
—**Andy Dufresne**, Shawshank Redemption

David

I (Chan) met a 19-year-old young man named David in a focus group in Tulsa, Oklahoma on a sunny day in April many years ago. Our research team at the University of Oklahoma was conducting research on the housing needs of people living with HIV. During the focus group, I watched David interact with the other participants. I was struck by David's engagement with others and their engagement with him. David was happy, articulate, and relational. Later, when I had an opportunity to visit with David, I learned my "happy" new friend had just found out he had tested positive for HIV. David told me that when he disclosed his condition to his parents, they kicked him out of their home. He was currently homeless, sleeping under a bridge.

When I was visiting with David, I couldn't make David's happiness and engagement with others fit within my training as a psychologist. Psychologists have been interested in understanding what is wrong with people for decades. David had so much "wrong" in his life, and yet he was happy, resilient, and navigating successfully. My 10-minute conversation with a homeless young man with HIV changed the course of my personal and professional life. How could he be so happy, centered, and focused on his future? He should have been devastated, depressed, and discouraged. The answer: David was applying the science of hope in his life. He was navigating toward his goals and rising hope in his life gave him the strength and the resilience to deal with tremendous adversities.

What is Hope?

Very few people know anything about the science of hope and the common understandings and usages of the word have failed us. Right now, how would you define hope? Write it down on a piece of paper. Save it and consider your definition while you read this book. Our definition of the word has totally changed during our years journeying deep into the science. We think your definition will change too.

The common use of the word "hope" in the English language has never fully captured its meaning in the research that has been done in the last twenty years. Webster's Dictionary simply gives hope a future orientation: "To desire with expectation of obtainment or fulfillment." The Oxford English Dictionary defines it as: "Grounds for believing that something good may happen." The dictionary definitions reflect the view of hope in the 1950s when early mental health researchers were putting only a future expectancy on the concept of hope.

Though the Judeo-Christian traditions were the first to identify hope as a positive virtue, many faith communities have made it simply about "life after death" or simply making "God" the definition of hope. We are both people of faith, but neither of us have ever heard a sermon or a pastor or rabbi fully articulate the research-based meaning of hope—the idea that hope is a verb involving action and the ability to change the future. Whatever definition of hope you just wrote down, we want to help people of all different belief systems and life experiences understand it in a way they have likely never experienced before.

Many good, kind people unknowingly often refer to "hope" when they really mean a wish. "I hope you have a great day." "I hope you have fun on your vacation." "I hope it doesn't rain tomorrow." We say things like that every day. But we are not really talking about hope. You may be asking, why is a statement about avoiding rain tomorrow not hope? Because the person saying it has absolutely no control over the weather. Why isn't "hoping" you have a great day actually hope? Because unless someone is managing your day they cannot ensure you have a great day. Why isn't "hoping" you have fun on your vacation hope? Unless someone is going on your vacation with you and in charge of your fun, they have no power over your vacation enjoyment. When we make any of these statements, we are just throwing out a wish for another person—not hope.

Even during the toughest times in life, well-intentioned friends make statements like: "I hope things get better for you" or "Everything is going to work out." Those statements are usually little more than wishes. We are all great "wishers" but not very good "hopers".

Hope is the belief that your future can be brighter and better than your past and that you actually have a role to play in making it better. Hopeful people embrace this truth with all of their being. Wishful people also believe their future can be brighter than their past, but they don't have any goals or critical thinking going on to help make their futures better. Hopeful people are willing to work for their better future. Wishful people aren't willing to do the work necessary to have hope and a better the future.

Psychologist Rick Snyder, the first "hope scientist", focused on the interaction of three concepts in defining hope—goals, pathways (waypower), and agency (willpower). Let's look at each element.

Goals

When we wake up in the morning, until we go to sleep in the evening, we are trying to achieve our goals. It is the essence of being human. These goals may be short-term, like getting to work on time, or they may be long-term, such as obtaining a college degree or a having a career in a particular field. When they get big, we often call them dreams. Goals may be crisis-oriented like staying alive in a forest fire or mundane like having a nutritious breakfast or dressing professionally for a meeting at work. The key is that your goals must be desirable enough to motivate you to action. Your goals must be things that excite you. It is also important to understand that goals are the focus for your "planned action."

Hope is not about impulsiveness or habit -- hope is about intention. Intention connects to what we believe, not what we know. We act based on what we believe not based on what we know. We know that too much sugar is not good for us, but we believe it will make us happy. We believe we deserve that extra cookie or that second serving of ice cream. Our goals connect to our beliefs about ourselves and about others. Goals can be domain oriented. Domain oriented goals are focused in one area of your life—like relationships or work or spirituality or children. And goals can be amoral. A rage-filled, desperate carjacker can be a person with high hope at a moment in time. His goal—stealing your car—may be a felony but it is nevertheless a goal. Goals we choose are not always healthy or moral. But the science is still applicable. The truth is, however, that moral goals will always produce better long-term outcomes and sustainable higher hope than goals that create victims, health consequences, or end you up in jail!

Pathways (Waypower)

Hopeful people can easily identify the pathways that will likely lead to their goals. Pathways are the roadmaps you have in your mind that allow you to begin the journey to the future. These roadmaps allow you to occasionally check your progress toward your goal. The hopeful person can identify multiple pathways toward a goal and plan alternative strategies when faced with barriers. Pathways always have a series of steps. Each time you take a step that moves you closer to a personal goal, your hope can rise. As soon as you are essentially "getting there" you are on a pathway to your goal. Pathways, like goals, can be moral or immoral. The car thief we mentioned above has an immoral goal—stealing your car. His pathway may include pulling a gun or a knife to get you out of your car. Once stopped or caught, his hope will drop fast because his goal and pathway are crimes and his high hope is not sustainable.

Most of this book will focus on sustainable hope—how we can choose moral, healthy goals and pathways and then sustain them through life's trials and challenges. We must remember, however, that high hope is never a constant. It is not linear. We have goals and we achieve them by finding pathways. Then, we have goals and we cannot achieve them and we must find new goals. Even the highest hope people sometimes struggle with low levels of hope as well. During great adversity in our lives, we often struggle to find hope. This is a constant process in our lives—goal setting, re-goaling, pathways and perhaps alternative pathways.

After we have identified a goal, and pathways to achieve a goal, the next piece is agency.

Agency (Willpower)

Agency is the motivational aspect of hope. It is often associated with cheerleaders, close friends, or mentors in our lives that spur us on to pursue our goals. Agency is a complex term used to describe your ability to dedicate mental energy (willpower) to begin and sustain the journey toward your goals. Mahatma Gandhi focused on the importance of willpower often. Gandhi said, "Strength does not come from physical capacity. It comes from an indomitable will." Author Dan Millman put it this way, "Willpower is the key to success. Successful people strive no matter what they feel by applying their will to overcome apathy, doubt or fear."

Willpower is limited each day. We each have a finite amount of it. Psychologists have found that willpower is connected to the glucose levels in our blood. Glucose here is not about eating more sugar, it is about what your body naturally produces. We will talk more about nutrition later. When you exert your willpower throughout the day you are also depleting glucose resulting in the experience of mental fatigue. Knowing that your willpower is limited during the day, it is easy to see how other areas of your life are impacted in the ways you respond to goal setting in the face of stressful situations that might deplete your energy. Maintaining motivation becomes key. Author Brian Tracy says it this way, "Willpower is essential to the accomplishment of anything worthwhile."

Your level of agency/motivation may depend very often on having cheerleaders and social support to pursue your goals and pathways. People who attend support groups for recovery or addiction often say that the group gives them the motivation to stay sober. This is about increasing their motivation to pursue their goal of sobriety or recovery. Being part of a strong social group, church, or athletic club often encourages people to pursue their goals. What is happening? Agency. Their willpower is increased or rejuvenated by having support in their lives as they pursue their goals.

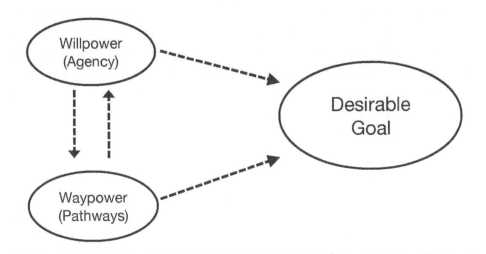

Rick Snyder loved to say hope means, "You can get there from here." He was acting as a cheerleader when he said it to people. Willpower and waypower produce the reality of hope: "You can get there from here." Now, there is a statement you can use that is not a cliché or a meaningless platitude. "You can get there from here" is not wishful. It is an aspirational statement that can motivate someone. After David was diagnosed with HIV and kicked out of his home by his parents, he had to set new goals and find motivation to pursue those goals. Then, he had to figure out pathways to those new goals and determine in his soul if he believed the statement was true—"I can get there from here."

Goals, Agency, and Pathways Are Like a Minivan

Think of goals, agency, and pathways as a minivan. For those with kids or grandkids, we all know the journey to load everything in the minivan for a trip. It is the minivan to hope. Goals are the destination for your journey. This could be a short or a complex cross-country journey. If you want to go visit friends or family, there are numerous routes. Like any journey, your goal requires a map that can provide the detailed pathways of the many different roads that lead to your goals. Like life, some pathways lead directly to the goal whereas others are perhaps more complicated. How many times have we achieved our goals only to look back and think, "There was an easier way!" Sometimes people don't have a map to help them choose the correct pathways to their goals and they get lost.

Agency is the engine in the van you use to navigate your pathways. Agency requires you to continuously stay tuned and replenish when you run low on fuel. We have to replenish the gas (agency) so our van can continue the journey toward our goals. We use the analogy of a van because we often have to carry our daily burdens on our journey. In real life, these are screaming children. But in the analogy, they are a lot of things. Our burdens can be the normal daily stress of responsibility and competing goals. They can be the attention-robbing force of trauma. They can also be physical or mental health challenges. Where do your burdens sit in your van of hope? For us, our childhood adversity is always on the journey with us. It never totally leaves the van. As people with high hope, we have learned strategies to put most of these burdens in the back of the van so their capacity to distract us on our journey is limited. If our burden is unmitigated or triggers us, it is likely sitting in the front seat detracting our attention through rumination, worry, regret, or other negative emotions. When our burdens are in the front seat, our attention gets diverted to things that don't matter in the context of our destination or goals. Healthy hope puts the burdens in the back of the van and always looks forward, not backward.

Both Pathways and Willpower Are Needed

Both pathways (waypower) and agency (willpower) are required for you to have hope. When you have a pathway to the goal but are not motivated to follow that pathway, you would be considered low hope due to your lack of willpower. On the other hand, you might have high willpower toward the goal you want to achieve but do not know how to get there—resulting in lower hope because you lack pathways. Is your goal to play in the NBA? If nerf basketball with your kids is a workout, there is probably no pathway to your goal. *Willpower without pathways is a wish.* We have already seen how often the word "hope" is used when we really mean a wish. Every day. People may look at you funny for a while when you start using words accurately until they too understand hope.

Some bypass the conversation about the importance of pathways altogether. But no amount of motivation can overcome a lack of pathways. Pathways need to exist for your goals to be accomplished. But what about, "Where there is a will, there is a way?" A great slogan but not always true. Ultimately, if no pathway is found, willpower will diminish over time and hope will suffer. When willpower dies, your goals usually die as well. Goals may need to be changed if there is truly no pathway. The NBA contract may have to give way to another dream. Let's consider a story about a dear friend, diagnosed with breast cancer, to illustrate the key pieces of hope—goals, pathways, and agency.

Ellen

Ellen was diagnosed with late stage breast cancer. Ellen was a high hope person in most of her life, but at 56, it was a devastating diagnosis. She was married with a son, and had a great job leading a national non-profit organization in St. Paul, Minnesota. She was a national leader in the violence prevention movement focused on addressing gender-based violence and abuse. But now she had to focus her mental energy on how to get the help she needed for breast cancer. Ellen didn't want to go from place to place for her diagnosis, treatment plan, and support system. She wanted to go one place. She quickly found she could go one place—called Cancer Centers of America. Cancer patients are flocking to Cancer Centers of America and similar wraparound services approaches, where all their services as are being provided under one roof. Ellen wanted to survive and overcome the devastating disease she faced. The first step for her was finding one place where she could "belong" and have a diagnosis and treatment plan that included integrated medical, mental health, nutrition, and relational support for herself and her family. The integrated treatment approach she developed with her multi-disciplinary team was a pathway to hope as she pursued her ultimate goal: Remission.

Ellen did not accomplish her ultimate goal. She died on January 6, 2012 surrounded by her family and close friends. But she taught us about hope during her journey through childhood adversity, battling discrimination in her advocacy for the LGBTQ community, championing social change for survivors of family violence, and navigating terminal cancer. When Michael Paymar, her colleague for so many years, eulogized Ellen he said, "If you want to change the world, if you want to change people, you have to do it with love in your heart. And she did." We honor Ellen as one of the first hope heroes you will see throughout this book.

The support being provided by wraparound services approaches for cancer patients in many health systems today increases a patient's *agency/motivation* as the patient navigates their *pathways*. *Willpower* helped sustain Ellen's *waypower* as she pursued the strength and support to continue her battle and pursuing her real goal—complete remission. She helped created many pathways for many women, men, and children in this country in her career. Even until her death, she determined to choose goals and pathways that would leave a legacy of love and advocacy for others.

Hope is Not Optimism or Self-Efficacy

When we give hope workshops, we are often asked how hope is related to optimism or self-efficacy. Several research studies have demonstrated the differences between hope and optimism. Optimism refers to the expectation that good outcomes will occur. While this future expectation is shared by both hope and optimism, hope includes both *pathways* thinking and the *willpower* to pursue selected pathways. Optimism is only the expectation itself. We all know optimistic people who always want to see the good or always want to expect the best. Some people are just naturally optimistic—others learn it over time. It is a great character trait but it is not always attached to the reality of a situation. Hope tends to increase optimism but optimism does not always increase hope. Sometimes optimism becomes false hope when there truly is no pathway to a goal. You are optimistic if you think the future will be better than the past. You are hopeful if you believe the future will be better than the past *and* you believe you have a role in making it so.

Helen Keller connected optimism and hope many years ago, when she said, "Optimism is the faith that leads to achievement. Nothing can be done without hope and confidence." A great quote but she was really talking about hope, not just optimism. Helen Keller was a doer, not just an optimist. Hope is the better focus than simply optimism. In our research, if hope rises, optimism rises as well. But the converse is not true. Optimism can rise while hope does not. Optimism will not sustain you if hope is not rising in your life.

Self-efficacy is different than hope or optimism. It refers to the confidence you have about your ability to pursue and attain a specific goal. It is a great character trait. But again, it may be based in the reality of your actual abilities or simply a belief in your abilities whether accurate or not. Confidence in your own abilities generally is a good thing and produces better outcomes than a low view of your abilities to pursue a goal or complete a task successfully. If you believe you can learn to speak Spanish as a second language, you are more likely to learn to speak Spanish. As you learn words and phrases, your sense of competency will rise. This does not necessarily mean you will learn to speak Spanish fluently. You will have to set goals and pursue those pathways diligently to become fluent. In the published research, hope tends to have a positive impact on self-efficacy but self-efficacy does not always increase hope. Hope as a verb (goals, pathways, and agency) will be a better approach to conversing in Spanish in two years than simply feeling good about your ability to learn Spanish.

We must aggressively pursue everything we want in life. Author Gavin deBecker in *The Gift of Fear: Survival Signals That Protect Us from Violence* borrowed from William Wordsworth in saying, "In ourselves our safety must be sought. By our own right hand, it must be wrought." The same is true of hope.

If David, living homeless with HIV, can be a high hope person, why can't you? If Ellen, even as she faced a terminal illness, could choose hope, why can't you? What is the excuse for not choosing hope? David and Ellen found hope and the research corroborates why it worked in their lives.

Every year we all create New Year's Resolutions, but seldom do they last the whole year long. Tennyson said, "Hope smiles from the threshold of the year to come, whispering 'It will be happier.'" But the truth is it *can* be happier and you have a role to play *if* that is going to be true. Hope is the idea that you have *goals* you desire to achieve, you can identify *pathways* toward the goals, and you can direct and sustain your *willpower* toward the goal and pathways necessary to reach those goals. This simple, yet powerful trilogy, now confirmed in hundreds of published studies, has become the science of hope.

The research has led us to follow three important research questions among vulnerable populations: (1) Does hope serve as a coping resource to stress? (2) Does hope predict adaptive outcomes? and (3) Can hope be improved and sustained? The answers are: Yes, yes, and yes.

The research is indisputable. Let's look more closely at why hope matters so much.

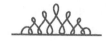

Chapter 3

Why Hope Matters So Much

"Hope is being able to see that there is light despite all the darkness."
—Bishop Desmond Tutu

Emeka

Emeka Nnaka watched the ball fly as the kick-off began the game. Emeka zeroed in on the returner as he caught the ball. The returner shed the first tackle, then ran through a block. He headed toward Emeka, coming full speed. Emeka wrapped him up. The sound of the collision reverberated throughout the entire stadium. Emeka made the tackle as he felt a stinging sensation all over his body and then fell to the ground. He did not feel his body hit the ground. It was the last time the 6-foot 4-inch 240-pound defensive end would ever play football. In June of 2009, at the age of 19, the Nigerian immigrant's career playing semi-pro football for the Oklahoma Thunder was over.

Emeka did not know why his body did not respond when he tried to get up. The entire stadium was silent. He was on the field for an hour and eighteen minutes before the ambulance arrived. He felt distant from the voices around him and people working on his body. As they rolled him off the field, he wanted to give a "thumbs up" as he had seen so many times from injured football players on television but he could not move his arms. Emeka's injury would leave him paralyzed for life. After weeks in the hospital, he began the long road through physical therapy and his argument with God—"Why me?"

I (Chan) met Emeka after he became a student at OU. He inspired me and quickly became one of my hope heroes. It was an honor to ask him to share his views about hope. He has faced one of the greatest blows imaginable in his life. As he looks back, Emeka says his biggest trial was his greatest blessing. Through his faith in God, he found the motivation to begin setting new goals and finding new pathways to his goals. Today, Emeka is a motivational speaker, life coach, and hope advocate. He has refused to let his injury define him. He began to see himself as a piece of coal that survived great amounts of pressure to become a diamond. Today, he says it clearly, "I am that diamond."

Today, Emeka is a graduate student studying human relations at the University of Oklahoma. What is his personal philosophy? "Hope is not a step in life, it is a stance." In one instant, his life changed forever when he suffered a spinal cord (neck) injury resulting in paralysis and a life restricted to a motorized wheel chair. However, Emeka decided to focus on gratitude that he was still alive. His life could have been destroyed. Instead, he is a beacon of hope to those around him. Emeka is emerging as a world class motivational speaker who shares his message of hope with others. His personal mission is to inspire, empower, and unite others in drawing the masterpieces of their lives regardless of their circumstances. He regularly speaks to middle and high school students, churches, community events, and organizations spreading the message of goals, pathways, and agency. His message is how hope can be learned and that we are all worthy of rising hope in our lives. Meet Emeka at www.emekannaka.com.

Emeka's journey shows us how hope has mattered in the life of a paralyzed, young, ambitious football player. The hope Emeka found has consistently been identified by researchers as the key determinant in helping children, adults, and families not only endure and survive, but flourish out of the most difficult circumstances. Emeka needs it. We all need it. This chapter will you provide with the scientific legitimacy that hope enjoys in the emerging psychological literature. Emeka's story is not an anomaly.

The research shows that people with high hope do better in life than those with low hope. High hope helps us overcome trauma better than low hope. High hope helps people deal with losing their ability to walk better than low hope. High hope helps people do better in surviving cancer than low hope. High hope helps people do better in school than low hope. High hope helps people make better employees than low hope. High hope helps people navigate their way through natural disasters better than low hope. Higher hope is better than lower hope.

Pandora's Box

In ancient Greek mythology, the story of Pandora provides a historic context of hope. It turns out that Zeus was angry with humans for stealing the ability to make fire. Zeus decided to punish man by creating Pandora, who had beauty, charm, and curiosity. Zeus, sending her to earth to be married, gave Pandora a beautiful box as a wedding gift but also with the instruction to never open the box. After the wedding and curious about the contents, Pandora finally opened the box. However, there were no diamonds, gold, or beautiful jewelry. Zeus had filled the box with all the terrible evils to plague human existence on earth. Out of the box flew the torments of mind, body, and soul. Poverty, disease, sadness, misery, pain, hate, and other maladies flew from the box to torment men. Pandora quickly shut the box but it was too late, all the contents had escaped save one—hope. Pandora finally released hope from the box to treat the wounds created by the torments. The seldom told part of Pandora's story reminds us that even in our darkest times, hope can endure.

Hope and Well-Being

Hope is an important psychological strength that has at least three important components. *First*, hope can buffer the effects of adversity and stress and serves as an important coping resource for both children and adults. *Next*, hope predicts adaptive thoughts and behaviors. Put simply, hopeful people have better outcomes connected to the way they think and behave. *Finally*, and most important to all of us, hope can be learned. Intentional strategies or interventions can move the needle on hope.

In every published study of hope, <u>every single one</u>, **hope is the single best predictor of well-being** compared to any other measures of trauma recovery. This finding is consistently corroborated with other published studies from top universities showing that hope is the best predictor for a life well-lived.

Hope has enjoyed a prominent role in the emergence of the positive psychology movement and its focus on understanding what makes a life worth living. For much of the 20th century, the field of psychology followed the medical model and focused on alleviating mental illness. Going all the way back to Freud, well-being in traditional psychology, has been the reduction of such things as depression, anxiety, or fear. Positive psychology introduced a new focus on well-being in trying to understand both happiness and the capacity to flourish. Prominent psychologists Martin Seligman, Christopher Peterson, and others developed a classification system of 24 character strengths (including hope) that are morally valued across cultures and contribute to our capacity as human beings to flourish. While all 24 character strengths have empirical support and do, in fact, contribute to our well-being; the character strength of hope is recognized as the best predictor of well-being. This line of research led Rick Snyder to write in referring to hope, *"All strengths are equal. Some strengths are more equal than others."*

We agree with Rick Snyder that it is time to declare, to everyone who will listen: The predictive power of hope in a person's life is greater than any other character strength.

Before describing some of our studies at The Hope Research Center at the University of Oklahoma, it is worth noting that today as we write this very sentence, there are over 2,000 published studies on hope. These studies consistently demonstrate the power of hope in the areas of education, work, health, mental health, social relationships, family, and recovery from trauma. Hope is no longer just a theory, hope is a science.

Adults and children with higher hope do better in navigating injuries, diseases, and physical pain. They score higher on satisfaction, self-esteem, optimism, meaning of life, and happiness. They perform better in sports even when abilities are equal. They excel at higher rates in academics from elementary to graduate school. In sports and academics, higher hope produces better results even when controlling for natural abilities. Studies to date have not found that men or women differ in their Hope scores. Our research has likewise not found any inherently different levels of hope in varying ethnic or minority backgrounds. Hope is accessible to all of us. Let's look at a few specifics.

Hope and Education

Hope can predict academic achievement from elementary school aged children through graduate school. The higher the hope of a child, the higher the daily attendance rate, the lower the tardiness rate, the higher the grades, and the better the test scores. In high schools, hopeful children are more selective in the courses they choose. In the language of hope, they are intentionally choosing <u>pathways</u> to their <u>goals</u>. Hopeful high school students have higher grade point averages, fewer absences, higher graduation rates, and higher college enrollment rates. One recent study found that hope is a better predictor of college grade point average than traditional placement tests and high school grade point averages. Hope also best predicts student retention and college graduation rates. Emeka is living proof of the power of hope in a young, paralyzed man who still outperforms and overachieves far beyond other students who have the use of both their legs, but do not share such high hope.

This truth has been identified in a great deal of research but is seldom connected to high hope versus low hope. David Brooks at the *New York Times* recently focused on research that has found that "social and emotional deficits can trump material or even intellectual progress." Brooks wrote of one program to help high school students get to college, "Schools in the Knowledge Is Power Program, or KIPP, are among the best college prep academies for disadvantaged kids. But, in its first survey a few years ago, KIPP discovered that three-quarters of its graduates were not making it through college. It wasn't the students with the lower high school grades that were dropping out most. It was the ones with the weakest resilience and social skills. **It was the pessimists**." But he missed the real name for it. It was not pessimism, it was kids with low hope. They look like *pessimists* but the real issue is hope.

While all this is great news and certainly a strong endorsement for hope, our nation is on the verge of a great tragedy. The Gallup organization conducts an annual hope and student engagement survey of close to one million students from middle school to high school. Less than one-half of all children report being hopeful. The remaining students report being stuck or discouraged. In fact, only one-half of the students reported being engaged with school and 21% reported being actively disengaged. While we can argue about funding shortfalls and teacher shortages, the most important and seldom discussed concern should be on the hope of our youth. We are losing the battle for hope. We are failing to build hope in the children of America.

We are ignoring the power of hope and its ability to produce highly motivated and successful children. Shane Lopez' research found students with higher hope perform a full Grade Point Average (GPA) higher than students with the same intellectual capacity that have lower levels of hope (14% higher GPA in high hope students). Higher hope produces an A, whereas lower hope produces a B in students with the same intelligence. This means students with higher hope, but a lower IQ, can outperform smarter students with lower hope. Rising hope is crucial to the future of education in America. We can debate the differences between public and private schools. We can debate the role of charter schools. We can argue about pay and benefits for teachers. We can demand nicer educational facilities. But the real issue in education today is the need for rising hope in the lives of our students.

Gallup Student Poll

Shane Lopez was the creator of the Gallup Student Poll (www.gallupstudentpoll. com) that now measures hope in students grades 5-12 in participating schools across the country. To date, Gallup has recorded more than 5 million completed student polls. The poll measures engagement, hope, entrepreneurial aspiration, and financial/career literacy. The results are consistent with all the research on hope.

Hopeful students are 2.8 times more likely to report excellent grades and 3.1 times more likely to agree that they do well in school. Higher hope students are 4.1 times more likely to be engaged in school and 2.2 times less likely to miss a lot of school. Schools need to create cultures of hope just like Sharp Memorial Hospital did. Sadly, many schools are not even measuring hope out of fear that their results will not be good. They are living into the saying that "ignorance is bliss." But with hope so predictive of long-term positive outcomes for students, this should be a priority everywhere. In the realm of hope, ignorance isn't bliss, ignorance is inaction. Only when we know that we have low hope can we begin to make concerted efforts to raise it.

Hope and Work

There is also emerging literature on hope and important workplace outcomes like performance, turnover, and job satisfaction. Hopeful employees set more goals and more complex goals. They are better at critical thinking and problem solving associated with the pathways dimension of hope. Hopeful employees are more energetic in their pursuit of goals. It is not surprising that hope is significantly predictive of workplace performance given that both are associated with goal attainment. Hopeful employees are more likely to experience success in goal attainment; they also report higher levels of job satisfaction and commitment to the organization. Hopeful employees tend to be more helpful to their coworkers and contribute more to high performing work teams. Hope is also a coping resource that produces lower levels of burnout. In fact, hopeful employees are more likely to be engaged in their work and approach new tasks with vigor. Hope is also associated with lower turnover.

Shane Lopez, in his work-related research, found that employees with lower hope, given the same amount of work in a day as employees with higher hope, will take longer to do the same amount of work. In one study, higher hope people finished the same number of tasks by 4 PM and lower hope people needed until 5 PM to finish the same amount of work. Employees with higher hope did their work 12% faster. These findings should have implications for how employers hire and train their employees. Employers should be looking for workers with higher hope in their lives and employers should be aspiring to increase hope in the lives of those that already work for them.

A recent economic study found that a hopeful employee contributed increased profits of approximately 21% to the company in comparison to an employee with low hope. Hopeful leaders in companies are more likely to be inspirational, visionary, and concerned with employee well-being. Comparatively, those leaders with lower hope are more transactional in their style and tend to rely on coercion to motivate employees. This is why employers should be measuring hope and cultivating it in the lives of their employees and supervisors. It could transform workplaces around the world. We will look at this again later when we talk about building hope-centered workplaces in this country.

Hope and Health

Hope has been studied in medicine and nursing for several decades. When hope is high, patients respond better to treatment, are more likely to engage in prevention strategies, and are more likely to comply with their health providers recommendations. These findings are consistent across studies in cancer treatment, spinal cord injuries, diabetes, HIV/AIDS, and rehabilitation with occupational and physical therapy.

Hope has also been studied in children suffering from chronic illness. Dr. Duane Bidwell and Dr. Donald Batisky were two of the first researchers to look at hope in children suffering from end-stage renal failure. They found higher hope in children through five pathways: 1) Maintaining their identity by participating in activities and relationships outside of diagnosis and treatment; 2) Realizing community through informal connections with others living with the disease; 3) Claiming power by taking an active role in setting goals, self-advocating, and monitoring their condition; 4) Connecting to spirituality through prayer and other contemplative practices; and 5) Developing wisdom and then finding ways to "give back" to others. They found that hope was highest when children had more of these pathways in their lives rather than only a few. They also found that when children felt they had a "team of support" they evidenced higher hope. When children could set goals of any kind and accomplish them, they did better in treatment.

Jerome Groopman's *The Anatomy of Hope* is a wonderful account of how patients with higher hope respond more positively to even aggressive and terminal forms of cancer. Likewise, Groopman describes patients with lower hope who struggle more to overcome treatable cancers than higher hope patients. Dr. Groopman, a professor at Harvard Medical School, has found that hope, desire, and expectation often provide the strength for cancer patients to find a pathway to remission and health in dealing with conventionally hopeless diseases and suffering. Biologically, Groopman argues that hope stimulates the release of internal painkilling molecules, giving cancer patients the energy to stick with treatment, and, ultimately, impacting clinical outcomes in otherwise "terminal" patients. We will see the tolerance of pain as a strong indicator of higher hope in many situations as we go deeper into the science. Let's look at two examples—one story about cancer and one about arthritic knees to see how hope made the difference.

Hope and Cancer

One story from Dr. Groopman's work with cancer patients is particularly compelling. More than 20 years ago, Dr. Groopman met Dan Conrad, a Vietnam veteran, diagnosed with a large cancerous mass that extended from his diaphragm all the way into his abdominal cavity. The mass was nearly a foot in diameter. The ultimate diagnosis was non-Hodgkin's lymphoma. Any chance for survival would require immediate and aggressive treatment. Dr. Groopman met with Dan and provided his diagnosis. Surgery was not an option—the cancer had spread too far.

Traditional chemotherapy was Dan Conrad's only chance but Groopman told him there was a new, experimental antibody treatment that he would like to try with the traditional chemotherapy. But Dan was unconvinced and decided to refuse chemotherapy. He told Groopman he felt his fate was inevitable. Groopman did not give up though. Even as Dan's health deteriorated rapidly, Groopman searched for the key to changing Dan's mind about treatment. Finally, the answer became clear—it was fear that was framing Dan's thinking. A fellow Vietnam veteran had been diagnosed with cancer, had submitted to chemotherapy, contracted pneumonia, and then died after seven terrible days of suffering. Dan witnessed every step of the journey and did not want to die like his friend. Once the fear was articulated, Groopman challenged Dan to just take one step at a time in the treatment process with the option of ending treatment at any time. Dan Conrad finally agreed to this approach. Set a *goal*: Treatment. Identify a *pathway*: One chemo treatment at a time.

Less than three months later, Dan was still alive after multiple rounds of chemo and radiation. Afterwards, he decided to have surgery to repair damage to his intestines caused by the largest tumor. Then, he underwent chemo for a second time and agreed to try the experimental antibody therapy that Groopman had recommended.

The experimental antibody therapy was only investigational but Dan became one of the first patients to receive this "monoclonal antibody" and it saved his life. Today, the experimental antibody therapy is FDA approved as Rituxan. Rituxan works by attaching onto lymphoma-forming immune cells, called B cells, causing the B cells to essentially commit cellular suicide, a process known as apoptosis. Dan Conrad's rising hope saved his life. It didn't happen overnight. Through his goals and pathways, one step at a time, he unknowingly opened the door for thousands of other cancer patients to later receive this life-saving experimental antibody.

Hope and Arthritis

The second study that Groopman profiled in *The Anatomy of Hope* was an early study looking at the so-called "placebo effect." In 2002, researchers at Baylor College of Medicine wrote up a study about pain relief and limb function in 180 patients suffering from arthritic knees. Two techniques were used on half the patients, one involving "lavage", which is simply putting saline solution into the knee, and the other involving "debridement", the removal of necrotic or infected tissue from the knee. But the other half of the patients underwent only a "sham" procedure where small cuts were made to mimic real surgery but nothing was done inside the arthritic knees. All patients were prepared for surgery in the same way and none of them knew which procedure they had endured. All patients received the same care after surgery and the nurses were not told what treatment each patient received. Stunningly, equal benefits, reduction in pain, were documented for patients who underwent the "sham" surgery and patients who underwent lavage or debridement—actual arthroscopic surgery.

The patients at the beginning of the arthritis study all knew they had a one-in-three chance of undergoing a placebo procedure but a two-in-three chance of having an actual procedure that might relieve pain and discomfort. This caused the researchers to hypothesize that all patients had higher expectations of benefits—*goals*—and, therefore, the willingness to choose this *pathway* toward reduction of pain. Billions of dollars spent every year on actual surgeries for such pain therefore were thrown into question in contrast with the benefit from the "placebo effect" created by increased hope in the patients that never even received the actual surgery. Rising hope reduced pain.

Hope and Diabetes

Families with children living with diabetes experience stress, fear, and uncertainty associated with sickness, emergency room visits, and nutritional management of a chronic, life-threatening disease. Several studies have found that hope-based intervention programs for parents can significantly reduce emergency room visits for their children with Type 1 diabetes. This research also demonstrates a significant reduction in the stress parents experience in the care of their children. But hope is important for the child as well. Research has consistently found that increasing a child's hope predicted better management of their blood glucose. Hope interventions helped increase the ability to pursue health-related goals and overcome obstacles to their diabetes care. When a child with diabetes has an increase in hope, they are empowered to manage their disease and pursue their dreams.

Hope and Mental Health

In mental health practice, hope is considered a critical protective factor that is required for recovery from both short-term and long-term illness. Studies have also shown that mental health patients can learn the science of hope and apply it successfully to improve outcomes. In one study, outpatients at a community health center were first taught hope-centered principles before entering their normal treatments. Compared to patients that did not learn these principles, the hope-educated patients showed significantly increased outcomes. In another study, female survivors of childhood incest were shown videos of hopeful narratives. A control group viewed a tape of nature scenes. Those who watched the hopeful narratives reported consistently higher Hope scores.

In research on bipolar disorder and depression, hope has also won the day. High hope helps people better navigate life with issues like bipolar disorder (Type I or II). They are more likely to navigate their way through other mental health issues as well including depression and schizophrenia. Across all therapeutic techniques, hope is considered one of the most significant contributors to the recovery from mental illness. The research demonstrated that setting and achieving goals increased hope among those with serious mental illness. In turn, this increase in hope was identified as the turning point in recovery by the patients, mental health professionals, and caregivers alike.

But what if someone eventually takes their own life due to depression or succumbs to major mental illness and never recovers? Does it mean hope did not make a difference? It does not. Hope is the single best predictor of physical, spiritual, and mental well-being even if eventually the deep pains of life, and particularly childhood trauma, do cut lives short at some point. We have often seen in our research that many with major mental health issues access high levels of hope to manage their difficulties and live successfully for many years even if a time comes when the consequences of their pain and trauma end their lives prematurely. This ability to make psychological adjustments is often correlated directly to their level of hope.

The research on hope indicates that hopeful children and adults experience superior adjustment to life experiences. Hopeful people learn how to "re-goal" or adjust their goals when they come up against unachievable goals. They adapt, making slight changes in their goals, to then successfully achieve their modified goals.

Hopeful people are better at self-regulating their emotions, thoughts, and behaviors as they pursue their goals in life. Hopeful people are also less likely to ruminate on their past and they experience reduced depression.

Seniors and Aging

Studies have also shown that hopeful thinking can be increased in seniors. In one study, a group of older adults who were experiencing depression learned how to improve their goal-setting priorities. Essentially, they were taught how to find pathways to their desired goals and given ideas for how to motivate themselves. A control group went through "reminiscence treatment" in which they recalled enjoyable previous experiences that took place during their younger years but were taught nothing else about hope. The seniors trained in hope-enhancing skills showed a significant reduction in depression compared to the control group based on self-reporting and objective behavioral markers. Hope matters at any age or stage of life.

Hope and Major Health Crises

Through major health crises, like Emeka's life changing football injury, we need the protective factor of hope. Along with all the other research we have cited, there is research in the areas of spinal cord injury, HIV/AIDS, and degenerative disorders that demonstrate the relationship between hope and positive outcomes. Emeka is quick to point out that his favorite hope quote is, by the late professor Dennis Sleebey, "Sometimes we have to lend hope to others, until they can find it for themselves." Emeka told us while he was in the hospital after his injury there were many people who would lend him hope.

During a health crisis, higher hope provides many coping benefits. Hope is based upon our ability to accurately appraise the reality of the crisis to set valued goals and find the means to achieve those goals. When faced with a major health crisis, it is natural to experience pain, anxiety and fear of the unknown, and even anger and despair when our goals are suddenly blocked. However, higher hope will allow us to navigate the crisis to set new goals and identify the pathways and options to remedy the situation. We must focus and pursue those components of hope (goals and pathways) that are in our

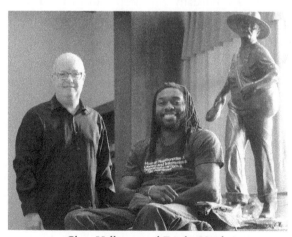

Chan Hellman and Emeka Nnaka

power to control. This will give us the ability to cope with psychological distress and adjust to the health crisis.

Emeka had a spinal cord injury and was paralyzed. This was his reality and as a result of his hope, he did not choose despair. As a hopeful person, he was faced with negotiating his life goals and ultimately was able to shift (re-goal) from being an elite football player to becoming a highly educated life coach and motivational speaker. He found his pathway through a graduate education at the University of Oklahoma and is seeing his dreams come true.

Emeka's story of hope has been documented time after time in the research. Terrible tragedy, pain, and difficulties can be overcome with high hope. The research proves it. *Hope is not a wish. Hope is measurable. Hope is malleable. Hope is action. Hope matters.*

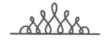

Chapter 4

Telling the Truth About Your Life

If a miracle happened, and you could have your life be exactly the way you want it, what would it be like? Your journey to higher hope begins with an honest appraisal of who you are, how you think about your life, what you want for yourself, and how you can get what you want.

—Psychologist **Rick Snyder**

You

You are writing your story right now. Throughout this book, you will see every chapter start with a story about hope. As you read each story, reflect on your own story. Are you truly satisfied with your life? Are there areas of your life where you have higher hope? Are there areas of your life where you have lower hope? Did things in your childhood steer you away from hope? Did painful things rob you of your ability to dream and pursue an amazing future for yourself? Maybe you aren't ready to share these answers with anybody else right now. Maybe you just need to process this personally and privately. We give you permission to be honest with yourself. This book will change your life, but only if you are willing to be honest about your own story.

Believing in hope is not a blind leap into the dark. The research confirms the reality and the power of hope. But the choice is still yours. First, you have to make *the choice to believe.* Second, you have to *make the choice to work for it.* We would love to see you start writing your story as you read this book. Maybe you can just start making some notes. Maybe you are ready to start telling a trusted friend part of your life story—not just the good parts version but more of the story that may have damaged your ability to hope or steered you away from being a hopeful person. What is your story about hope in your life? Maybe you live with a high level of hope most of the time. Maybe you need greater hope in your life. As we saw with Emeka, you can live with high hope and then some kind of trauma, adversity, or challenge can invade your life and threaten your ability to be hopeful.

Trauma, Adversity, and the Challenges of Life

One of the key themes of this book will be the importance of being honest about trauma, adversity, and the challenges of life you may have experienced. We shared a little bit of each of our stories in the Introduction. We will share the rest of our stories later. Trauma, the bad things we endure, negatively impacts our level of hope. Untreated and unaddressed trauma can cause long-term damage mentally, emotionally, spiritually, and physically. Here is the best definition of trauma to use going forward toward hope. *Trauma results from an event, series of events, or set of circumstances that are experienced by an individual as physically and emotionally harmful or threatening.* While there are many ways to define trauma, most definitions come close to this and focus on situations where someone has no control over what is happening to them or those around them.

Dr. David Lizak says fear is at the core of trauma. Fear is at the core of trauma symptoms and post-traumatic stress disorder (PTSD). Bessel van der Kolk says trauma gets trapped in the body. It is not just a mental issue. It becomes a physical issue as well. PTSD is a mental health condition that is triggered by a terrifying event but then can play itself out in the body. Trauma occurs primarily when we are in a situation where fear takes center stage. This covers trauma from fires, tornados, hurricanes, car accidents, sexual assault, domestic violence, child abuse, death of a loved one, major illness, bullying, poverty, community violence, and any other similar types of situations. The good news though is that rising hope reduces the impacts of these types of traumatic experiences. But we must learn to talk about the bad stuff and then engage in physical and mental efforts that help us release trauma from our body. If trauma is part of your story, practice telling it to someone you trust even as you read this book.

The vast majority of human beings have suffered trauma, adversity, or challenges in various forms. Dealing with it well is part of the pathway to hope—but you have to understand it and how it is impacting you, mentally and physically, before you can deal with it. We will talk much more about trauma later in the book but keep the definition above in mind as you reflect on your story. Psychologist Barbara Frederickson in her book on the power of positivity says we all have a choice whether we will languish or flourish. But we also need to know whether we are languishing or flourishing first—before we can decide what to do about it. Flourishing is not just about mental processes. It is about physical processes too. You cannot just sit and talk your way out of trauma. There is much more involved and you will need to get out of the chair or off the couch for trauma and "stuckness" to truly end up in the rear-view mirror.

The Survival Window

Fires have become common place, annual events in drought-ravaged California. In 2017, again, thousands evacuated to makeshift centers where Red Cross volunteers and many others tried to give comfort and hope. Hope, though, was in short supply as many felt the helplessness that often accompanies a natural disaster that is beyond the power of anyone to control.

As the Santa Ana winds blew and the fires raged, many on the West Coast lost their homes. The trauma was profound even for those watching on the news as horses caught fire in corrals at San Luis Rey Downs in North San Diego County and could not be saved. Firefighters battled to save everyone and everything they could, but people died and hundreds of homes burned to the ground.

News stories on every fire reported "zero percent containment" for weeks. The trauma to hundreds of thousands was real and nothing could prevent it. On social media, many posted of the terror of immediate evacuation as they grabbed only a few personal items and rushed away from burning hillsides and 80 mph winds. KTLA reported one fire increasing from 400 acres to 3,500 acres in less than three hours fueled by dry brush and raging winds. It was a time of terror, trauma, and flight.

As the Thomas fire in Ventura and Santa Barbara Counties still burned, the largest in the history of California, Rev. Dana Worsnop, a pastor in Ventura, decided to preach on hope. She acknowledged that for many there was no hope right now. They just have this "unsettled feeling you get when something like this has happened." "I didn't say to folks, 'Let's all just be hopeful now.' I said, 'I believe hope and grace and possibility still exist,'" Worsnop said. "You don't have to be hopeful right now. Know that it will return. Your sense of hope will return."

It was not yet a time for hope. Hope would come later, after the terror, after the trauma. After the devastating, heartbreaking loss of lives and homes—lifetimes of memories and mementos gone—everyone "hoped" for an end to the fires. They hoped for word that their house was spared. They hoped to find their pets. But this was not really hope. They were wishes. Residents had no power over the outcomes.

We call this the *survival window* when your focus is not on hope. When a loved one dies, it is a time of grief and loss. When the diagnosis is bad, it is a time of shock. When adversity slams into our lives, there is a window of time when we simply must struggle to survive. If someone tries to push toward rising hope in those moments, we will resent them and recoil as we process the heartbreak, pain, or loss. Dana Worsnop did not minimize the survival window in her sermon but she challenged people to still believe that hope would rise again.

We are not advocating a Pollyanna approach to hope. Nobody is hopeful all the time. We should not even aspire to be. To be fully human, we need to experience the vast range of human emotions in our life. There are times when we experience adversity, stress, and trauma and it is *natural and healthy* to experience the range of negative human emotions -- rage, despair, fear, grief, or regret. What is important is to become mindful of the experience and the emotions. However, as we allow the intensity of the negative emotions to run their course during the survival window, we need proven coping resources like hope to help us navigate back toward well-being. In fact, being hope-centered means that you have nurtured the psychological strength of hope so that when the adversity comes, and it will, that you will ultimately be resilient to the pain and able to re-center yourself on the power of hope.

The Choice to Believe

If we are going to overcome the adversities of life, however, we must eventually make a choice to believe that hope is our goal. Wishful thinking out of terrible struggle will not get us to hope. Hoping for the end of wildfires was wishful thinking. The fires of California each year remind many of the difference between hope, focused on things you have some control over, and wishful thinking, things you desire yet cannot control. In Hurricane Katrina, the people of the Louisiana and the rest of the Gulf Coast, experienced the same reality in a different type of natural disaster. During times when we lack control or any power to change things, is not the time for goal setting and pathways. But it must return and we must embrace, again, our definition of hope.

*Hope is the **belief** that a thriving future is possible and you have the power to make it so.* As we have seen, Rick Snyder focused on the interaction of three concepts—goals, pathways (waypower), and agency (willpower). Once we understand each element of the science of hope, we can start building it into our lives like the rebuilding of a home after a forest fire or hurricane. But the first step is still belief. You have to believe it exists or can exist again if it has been lost.

Not everyone has always believed in the power of hope. Plato called hope a "foolish counselor." The Greek philosopher Sophocles said human suffering was prolonged by hope. Not until the Jewish Torah was hope seen as a good thing. The Judeo-Christian tradition elevated hope to the equivalent of faith and love in the virtues of human beings. But as recently as Nietzsche, hope has been considered bad. Nietzsche called hope "the most evil of evils because it prolongs man's torment." Even one of the most famous founders of our country, Benjamin Franklin did not believe hope was real. Benjamin Franklin said that anyone who lives on hope will "die fasting." Ben Franklin was wrong. You have to choose to believe in it, then you have to work for it.

The Choice to Work for It

If you don't have high hope, are you willing to work for it? Thomas Fuller said, "Nothing is easy to the unwilling." Are you willing to take a close look at your life? Are you high hope in one area of your life and low hope in another? Each of our lives have different domains—Academics, Work, Family, Health, Fitness, Spiritual, Social, Romantic, to name a few. You may be high hope in one area and low hope in another. Now, we will ask you to think about your level of satisfaction in each of those domains before we dive deeper into the science of hope. This will help you see which areas of your life can benefit most from a boost in hope.

Let's take a quick look at areas where you are or are not satisfied with your life, these will be great places to apply the science of hope and create goals and pathways so the science can change your life.

Your answers to these questions will help you articulate your own story, decide if you are languishing or flourishing, and then help you identify where you need rising hope.

Domains of Life

For most of us, the important domains of our life include personal relationships, education, career and work, spirituality, family, finances, mental and physical health, and recreation and fitness. These individual domains can have different individual Hope scores. In the back of the book, we include some sample domains of hope you

LIFE SATISFACTION QUESTIONNAIRE

Directions: Consider each statement below in terms of how you have felt over the past year. Use the rating scale below to fill in the blanks in each statement.

Very Dissatisfied	Somewhat Dissatisfied	Neither	Somewhat Satisfied	Very Satisfied
1	2	3	4	5

1. I am _____ with my intimate relationship (spouse/significant other).

2. In my relationships with my family (parents, siblings, children), I feel _____.

3. I am _____ with my friendships in my life.

4. I am _____ with the work I do (in or outside the home).

5. As I think about my work/career achievement, I feel _____ so far.

6. I am _____ with the level of education I have attained.

7. I am _____ with my financial situation.

8. In terms of my ability to meet future expenses, I am _____.

9. I am _____ with my spiritual life.

10. I am _____ with my level of physical fitness.

11. I am _____ with the aspects of my appearance I can change.

12. I am _____ with the status of my health.

13. I am _____ with my emotional stability.

14. I am _____ with my recreational life.

15. I am _____ with my ability to be honest with others about past trauma in my life.

can measure in your life. The questionnaire above, however, attempts to just give you a quick screen of where you might be high hope or low hope.

People who answer the questionnaire with mostly 3's spend time mostly in the doldrums of marginal hope. People living with a lot of 1's and 2's have quite a bit of discontentment and therefore very low hope. People living with 4's and 5's tend to be fairly satisfied with their lives. Look at how you just rated yourself. Do you have areas of your life that need rising hope? Don't forget about your ratings. In the next chapter, we will measure your overall hope in your life. Later, we will talk about ways you can boost hope in your life—especially in the areas where hope is lowest.

You may be high hope in some areas of your life and low hope in others. You may be in a survival window right now experiencing the profound impact of loss, heartbreak, or adversity of some kind and hope may need to come later. But all of us likely have areas where we really would like Rick Snyder's "miracle" to happen. Rising hope is that miracle. It just takes hard, personal work for the miracle to happen. Let's go find the miracle.

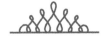

Chapter 5

Hope Should be Measured Everywhere

"Hope is actually something we create. It's not something that magically appears from an outside source. We each have within us the capacity to generate hope. It's critical that we be absolutely intentional about nurturing hope in our lives and the lives of our children. Don't let the bad news in the world be your undoing. You can take charge of hope."
—Naomi Drew

Rick Snyder

Rick Snyder, the first hope scientist, appeared on Good Morning America in 2000 to conduct a live experiment showing and measuring hope in action. He brought with him a cold pressor tank. A cold pressor tank uses ice water to assess pain tolerance. Rick knew a lot about pain tolerance. He suffered from chronic pain for many years in his life. Rick challenged Charlie Gibson, the host of GMA, the medical expert, Tim Johnson, and Tony Perkins, the meteorologist, to submerge their right fists into the cold-water tank for as long as they could stand it. Tony Perkins pulled out first—shaking his hand hard, trying to get feeling in it again. Charlie Gibson and Tim Johnson became extremely competitive and vowed to keep their arms submerged through the entire segment. Tim Johnson finally gave up just as the segment ended and they went to a commercial break. Charlie Gibson held on into the break.

When they came back from the commercials, Charlie Gibson was declared the winner but asked Rick Snyder what the contest had to do with hope. Rick told him the research on hope had found that hopeful people consistently tolerate more pain than their less hopeful counterparts. Then, Rick revealed to the national audience of GMA that Charlie, Tim, and Tony had taken a standardized hope test prior to the show and their Hope scores had accurately predicted the order in which each one would call it quits from the cold pressor tank. Charlie had the highest Hope score, Tim had the second highest Hope score, and Tony, the weatherman with no control over the weather, had the lowest Hope score of the three men.

Higher hope isn't just good in all the areas we have talked about so far. Research has found that hopeful people tolerate pain twice as long as those who are less hopeful. You can measure it by submerging your fist or entire body in a tank of ice cold water, or you can take the Adult or Children's Hope Scale with a pen and piece of paper. Your call.

At about the same time that Chan met David, the high hope, homeless, HIV positive, 19-year old, he was asked by Sharon Gallagher of the Tulsa Area United Way to present a 15-minute discussion on outcome assessment to 60 executive directors of United Way partner agencies. This meeting was chaired by Desiree Doherty, the Executive Director of the local child abuse prevention agency. At the end of his brief presentation on outcomes and the role of his research center, Chan was handing the microphone back to Desiree and made the offhand statement, "…and I've become interested in researching hope." Desiree was silent for several moments when she finally said, "You can't measure hope. You can't measure what we actually do with our families."

Chan leaned back and responded for the entire room to hear, "I can measure anything." Desiree, though doubtful, invited Chan to begin working with her agency, and now every child abuse and neglect prevention program in Oklahoma is measuring hope. The results are guiding social services programs in how to improve the lives of families and keep children safe. Desiree has become one of the biggest proponents of the power of measuring and then increasing hope.

The Adult Hope Scale

The Adult Hope Scale consists of 8-items designed to measure an individual's overall hopeful disposition. Rick Snyder developed the scale to measure both agency and pathways thinking toward goals. Four items reflect the agency (willpower) for past, present and future goals. Four items reflect the pathways (waypower) or mental roadmaps toward goal attainment. While subscale scores can be computed for both agency and pathways, adding scores from the eight items will represent your total Hope score.

Hope does not need to be ambiguous or vague. You can know your current hope level based on knowing your level of willpower and waypower. The Adult and Children's Hope Scales have now been administered to thousands of children and adults and are scientifically valid.

As we touched on earlier, there are also measures for specific domains of life, such as Work, Relationships, Health, etc. We like both the individual and the global measures of over-all hope in one's life. However, the global measures (looking at a person's entire life) tend to produce better outcomes than specific areas. The Hope Scale we are using here measures overall or "global" hope in your life. In the back of the book, we give you specific domains scales so you can measure hope in various areas of your life.

With this scale, we are not measuring optimism. We are not measuring resiliency. We are not measuring self-esteem. We are measuring hope. And the sooner we measure hope the better. It can serve as a baseline against your progress when you finish reading this book! It can also help you begin to think about your life in the context of hope.

So, first we measure it, then we score it. Then, we have a baseline for the rest of your life. Lean in. Don't try to manipulate the answers. Give the rating to each section that first comes to your mind. Don't over think it. Just rate each statement as honestly as you can and do it as soon as you read it.

You can do it below or you can go to www.hopescore.org. The benefit of doing it online is that our program scores your entries for you. We recommend measuring it at least once a year and maybe more if your circumstances of life change significantly. You can also measure individual domains in your life if you reach out to us and ask for our special domains worksheet. You can chart hope with your spouse or children as well. It is simple and straightforward. You can measure it below or you can pause your reading and go online now.

Instructions: Read each item carefully. Using the scale below, please select the number that best describes you.

Understanding Your Hope Score—Hope in Action

The Hope Scale has been administered to tens of thousands of people across the country and around the world. This is what makes norming possible. Scores of 40 or

THE ADULT HOPE SCALE

Directions: Read each sentence carefully. For each sentence, please think about how you are in most situations. Using the scale shown below, please select the number that best describes **YOU** and put that number in the blank provided. There are no right or wrong answers.

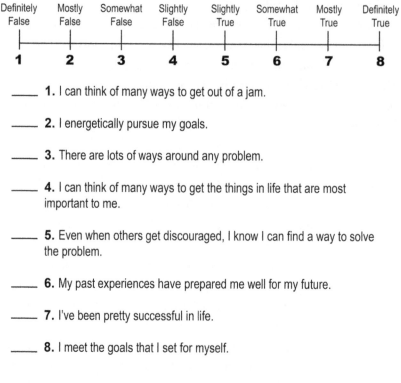

Definitely False	Mostly False	Somewhat False	Slightly False	Slightly True	Somewhat True	Mostly True	Definitely True
1	2	3	4	5	6	7	8

_____ **1.** I can think of many ways to get out of a jam.

_____ **2.** I energetically pursue my goals.

_____ **3.** There are lots of ways around any problem.

_____ **4.** I can think of many ways to get the things in life that are most important to me.

_____ **5.** Even when others get discouraged, I know I can find a way to solve the problem.

_____ **6.** My past experiences have prepared me well for my future.

_____ **7.** I've been pretty successful in life.

_____ **8.** I meet the goals that I set for myself.

Notes: The **Agency** subscale score is the sum of items 2, 6, 7 & 8; the **Pathways** subscale score is the sum of items 1, 3, 4 & 5. **Hope** is the sum of the four **Pathways** and four **Agency** items. Scores can range from a low of 8 to a high of 64.

Agency Score _____ (Add items 2,6, 7, and 8)

Pathways Score _____ (Add items 1,3,4, and 5)

Total Hope Score _____ (Agency Score + Pathways Score)

above put you in a hopeful category. Scores above 48 bump you up to a higher level of hope. Scores of 56 or higher make you a high hope person. Scores below 40 put you in a low hope category. Don't panic quite yet if you have low hope right now. It just means you have work to do. Our guess is that this will not surprise you. It might be you lack willpower, it might be you lack waypower, or it might mean you lack both. Fret not. There is a pathway to increasing willpower and waypower. If you are low in willpower (agency), you need to focus on how to surround yourself with people that can encourage and support you. If you are low in waypower, you need to connect with people to help you think strategically about ways to overcome obstacles and achieve your goals. If you are low in both, this book may be a wake-up call to a much more complicated journey toward higher hope that we discuss throughout the rest of this book.

Measuring Hope in All Adults

Hope not only *can* be measured as you just saw by taking your own score, it *should* be measured. It can be a barometer for our personal lives and a guide for agencies trying to help those impacted by trauma, abuse, or adversity of some kind. It can be used by *any* employer or business that is truly interested in the health and wellness of its employees.

If employees with higher hope are more productive than employees with lower hope, why isn't every company measuring hope? If high hope helps people navigate their way through difficult times more than low hope, why aren't we measuring it in every type of social and human services program? If people with high hope do better through all forms of cancer, why aren't cancer treatment centers measuring it? If high hope is better than lower hope in dealing with heart disease, diabetes, liver disease, and autoimmune disorders, then why aren't medical facilities and doctors' offices measuring it? If higher hope is better through natural disasters like fires and hurricanes, then why aren't we measuring it in disaster relief efforts? If higher hope serves adults and children better through divorce, why aren't court systems measuring it to see if their processes are producing higher hope and therefore less damage to children and adults? If students with high hope do better than those with low hope, why isn't every school in the country using the Gallup Student Poll to measure hope?

The truth is that many institutions and organizations don't want to know whether they are producing rising hope. Schools would have to answer to parents and funders if they were not increasing hope. Businesses would have to change their approaches if employees were not experiencing rising hope. It would impact retention efforts and perhaps even compensation levels. If social service organizations were not increasing hope, funders might pull out. Some might not want to know the truth about rising or falling hope. But it is our earnest desire to see measuring it become standardized throughout the culture and economy.

Rising or falling Hope scores can help social service providers develop strategies for improving services and support. Churches and synagogues should be increasing hope and if they are not, benchmarking hope levels can guide vision casting, planning, and programming. Rising or falling Hope scores of employees in a business, can help guide employee assistance programs and corporate wellness efforts. If hope is more predictive than standardized tests for measuring success in school, then we should be requiring it to be measured in every school district. This is the beauty of hope. You can measure it for yourself or you can measure it in a program or organization. Measuring it then serves as a tool, quantifying both pathways and agency, to guide policies and programs.

Hope Rising should be the story of our lives. Organizations, schools, and businesses of every kind should be measuring it as an indication of morale and well-being. If you are a leader and your business or organization is not causing hope to rise in the lives of those who work for you, you are failing your employees. You cannot sustain success in virtually any business, no matter how good your business model, unless your employees have high or at least increasing hope.

Case Studies to Better Understand Hope

More than fifteen years ago, Rick Snyder profiled four patients in *Making Hope Happen* as he was describing profiles of hope and what they could tell us about Hope in Action. We include all four in their entirety here:

Darcy—Ready to Quit: High Willpower, Low Waypower
Darcy announced that she was quitting her doctoral program. She had dreamed of being a clinical psychologist since she was an undergraduate. "I worked so hard to get good grades," she said through tears. "I even took a special course to do well on the entrance exams. I've done everything right to get into this program, and now I'm failing two of my courses. I just don't know what to do except quit."

"Tell me about which courses are hard for you."

"Biology and pharmacology are the hardest ones." She blew her nose and dabbed her tears. "Honestly, the professor and other students seem to be speaking a language I've never heard. This program is so much harder than anything I have done before, and I'm beginning to think I made a mistake coming here."

"You've had other difficult courses in the past." "Tell me how you managed to get through those."

"They were nothing like these." She wadded her tissue and continued. "Sometimes I think I don't have the background for this work, but when I had problems before I usually discussed them with the teacher."

"What's stopping you from doing that now?"

"I guess I don't want to seem stupid. It just didn't seem appropriate to do that in graduate school. But I don't want to quit. I am determined to get this degree, so I'll just have to put my pride aside and see what help I can get."

Darcy had been a highly motivated undergraduate student, but the small college she attended had not offered her enough challenges. She was not used to finding work difficult, and in the face of impending failure, she experienced anxiety and self-doubt. Her highly emotional state prevented her from seeing solutions, and her impulse was to give up. Talking it over with her advisor, and identifying the specific problems, helped Darcy to see that the total picture was not as bad as she thought at first. Once she could overcome her emotional reaction, she could find ways, with the help of an advisor, to prepare for these difficult courses.

The advice she received from her advisor was focused on her waypower, her pathways to her goals, and helped her think of ways to navigate toward her goals. So, if you are low in waypower in your score, this is the focus area for you. How can you learn to think about ways to overcome obstacles and challenges? Who can help you think through strategies when you are unable to come up with those ways to overcome? If you are advising someone with similar challenges in their life, have them take the Hope Scale and then decide if the problem is related to willpower or waypower.

Larry—Words, Words, Words: Low Will, High Ways
As a college student, Larry became engrossed in philosophy, reading all the major writers and memorizing their wisdom. His professors believed he had great potential because of his brilliant class debates. But when it came to putting his ideas into writing, Larry lacked the energy necessary to do the work. Recognizing that his academic record was riddled with incomplete and dropped courses, he came to the counseling center for help.

The first session with Larry was a struggle to help him focus on what had brought him for counseling. Instead, he wandered into intellectual discussions relating philosophy to psychology and avoiding the real issue that concerned him—his academic failure. What he was finally able to reveal was that he really preferred to talk about his ideas rather than write about them. He found the discipline of writing to be tedious and uninteresting, while discussions with other people were stimulating and exciting.

"All the way through high school my teachers thought I was great. I have a lot of good ideas, but I just don't seem to have the motivation to write about them."

"When you are trying to put your ideas into writing, what thoughts do you have?"

"It just seems like too much work. I get tired and tell myself I can do it later. But when later comes there's always something I'd rather do that's more fun and not so hard."

Larry's real issue was not pathways. His real issue was willpower. He never developed the ability to motivate himself to overcome challenges that might get in his way. If you take the Hope Scale, and identify your issues to be around agency/willpower, it means you need to think about what inspires you so you can find the motivation to do what is needed. Likewise, if you are working with someone and you determine they are low in agency/willpower, it should lead to conversation about inspiration and what excites them rather than a conversation about pathways.

Shawna—Missing Out on Life: Low Will, Low Ways
Shawna spent her high school years like she had all her other years in school—on the fringes of what was happening. She was neither popular nor unpopular, but had a small circle of girlfriends, who were very much like her. Shawna's grades were average, mainly C's and B's, and she rarely attracted the attention of her teachers. She occasionally thought about joining a club or trying out for spirit squad, but she never felt enough "pep" to do those things.

One course Shawna did enjoy was Technical Literacy where she learned word processing and various business skills. As a result of this course, Shawna decided to become a secretary after she graduated. She thought that working for a doctor or lawyer might be interesting, but she did nothing to get that type of job. Instead, Shawna applied for work through a secretarial service, believing that one of the temporary jobs would lead to permanent employment.

Almost immediately Shawna was sent to work for an insurance agent who had a small office. His secretary was on maternity leave and he needed an energetic and resourceful individual to take her place. When Shawna realized she would be alone in the office, she was apprehensive about her new duties. Her employer was patient, however, and showed her various forms and reports he needed typed. As the first day drew to a close, Shawna's exhaustion was openly visible. Her work was slower and she heaved deep and frequent sighs. Concerned her employer asked her if she would be able to do the amount of work there was in his office. Shawna had serious doubts.

The next day Shawna called her agency, telling them she was ill and could not go back to the insurance company. Over the next months, she worked at a series of jobs, never enjoying any of them enough to seek permanent employment. With the end of each temporary job, Shawna felt a loss of self-confidence and a desire to change her life. She saw her friends from high school get interesting jobs, marry, and have children. Her life was racing by, and Shawna's low hope was preventing her from catching a ride.

Shawna preferred to play it safe and take no risks rather than risking failure. She did not know how to shine and when she did have a chance to shine, her low agency/willpower wiped out her ability to find a pathway to success. If you are like Shawna, you are facing challenges around both key elements in the Hope Scale. You are a low hope person and addressing it will take some very conscious efforts around willpower and waypower. Don't give up though. This book can be your pathway. If you are working with a low hope person, don't give up on them. Hope can rise. Willpower and waypower can increase, usually in small increments at first. Very often, low hope is connected to trauma in life. Low hope people may not know why they have low hope but beginning to talk about their childhood and adult experiences ("What happened to you?" versus "What is wrong with you?") can help start the process to rising hope.

For the last scenario, let's look at a high Hope score person. Rick Snyder shared one such example in his workbook on hope. Let's see how high hope looks.

Matt—From Making Coffee to Making Recordings: High Will, High Ways
Ever since the family could remember, Matt had loved music. When he was a baby, he had his music box, as a toddler he beat on pans as drums, in grade school he played the trumpet, and as a teenager his boom box was blaring constantly. When, at fourteen years old, Matt was hired to work the light and sound panels for a children's theater company, his future goals were set. Matt knew he had to work in the music industry, no matter how he got there.

Because he knew what he intended to do with his life, Matt cared little for his high school classes. He began skipping school in his junior year, spending his time instead at a local recording studio. The older artists and engineers taught Matt a great deal about making records, and by Matt's senior year he knew he wanted to drop out of school. His parents understood his love of music and, while they would have preferred that he finish high school, they allowed him to attend a training program for recording engineering instead.

Once in the training program, Matt worked hard and graduated at the top of his class. He knew he was on the right track. His new credentials were valuable, but the challenge was finding work. The music industry is difficult to break into, but Matt was up to the task. With a small allowance from his parents to help him as he got started, he found work as a "gofer" in a well-known recording studio. He was asked to go for coffee, to answer the phones, and even to scrub the bathrooms, in exchange for rubbing elbows with the top-name musicians.

As the months and years went by, Matt was allowed to engineer occasional songs, getting an opportunity to show what he could do. Matt was very good; a few musicians began to ask for him. In time, his reputation grew until his work was in demand by well-known artists. Matt had the ability to understand the sound console, he could translate their vision into beautiful music. As the years went by, Matt made less coffee and more music, and today he is a foremost recording engineer with several gold and platinum records to his name.

Matt's journey is like other people that know what they want to do as children or young adults and can pursue those dreams without being sidetracked by trauma, abuse, or other obstacles. He was high willpower and high waypower. If you are high hope from childhood forward, you are blessed. In our work, we don't often see large numbers of people with high Hope scores throughout their lives, but it is still helpful to see what high hope looks like even in someone that never attended college or graduate school. This was not Matt's dream and his goals and success in life did not require college or graduate school.

Rick Snyder's stories—Darcy, Larry, Shawna, and Matt—are great retrospective views of the science of hope but none of them understood what was happening to them at the time nor did they understand what they could do about it to change their destinies. It would have helped them to know that hope was measurable, measure it, and then be able to see what they needed to do about it. We are now teaching children and adults to be aware of the science and know what to do to produce rising hope. Some of the stories are inspiring but not every story is a happy ending. Choices matter.

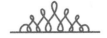

Chapter 6

Measuring Hope in Children and Teens

"It is easier to build strong children than to repair broken men."
—Fredrick Douglass

Nora

Nora remembers the day her mom died. She was 12. Her mom had been sick for two years. Everyone said her mom shouldn't be dying from it—early stage Alzheimer's Disease. No one knew why. Her mom grew up in a healthy, happy home. No brain trauma. No violence. No abuse. Why was it happening? Why this cruel cosmic joke? Why was God allowing her mom to fade away like this?

Nobody noticed at first. There were little clues when Nora was 7 years old. Her mom couldn't remember where she had parked her car after hours of fun shopping at the mall. Nora learned to pay attention to details like that for her mom. Then, a name forgotten at church. Someone her mom knew well. Nora and her dad both learned to say the name before it became embarrassing for her mom. Then, her mom needed more help. Her dad would leave notes to remind her mom what to do on any given day. Doctors prescribed Aricept, an Alzheimer's drug, which seemed to slow the progression of the disease. Her mom was scared at first but as the realization set in that there was no cure, her mom settled in to the reality of the journey ahead.

In the later stages of the journey, Nora tried to remember only the happy times—when her mom remembered her, when her mom loved her, cheered for her, and spent countless hours with her. She remembered the vacations her dad planned even though they didn't really have the money. Her dad said, "Memories are worth more than our credit card payments." Truth. The day soon came when her mom couldn't travel and she couldn't recognize anyone. Then, there were days when Nora's mom called out to her dead grandmother and grandfather. A minister said her mom had "one foot on each side of eternity."

The day her mom died was a day Nora will never forget. Her dad told her that it was okay if she stayed home from school. The hospice nurse said that her mom's breathing was coming slowly with long pauses between the heaving of her chest. It meant the time was short. When her mom's eyes were closed and her mouth was open, Nora watched her from the doorway of the room. It looked like she was already dead. She and her dad prayed with her mom. Her mom gave no indication that she knew anyone. Her dad finally prayed that God would end the suffering. Hours later, her dad's prayer would be answered.

Nora's grief was unbearable. Her dad could offer her little comfort for months. He became dark and seemed lost in his loneliness. Nora tried to bury herself in school and sports. Some days she felt normal. It was nighttime when she struggled the most—when her mom didn't come to tuck her in or pray with her or tell her a story. The months dragged by. Her dad took her to counseling and eventually her dad agreed to join her in counseling together. Finally, they wept in each other's arms in the counselor's office. They would cling to each other. They would begin, together, to take one step at a time toward a future without her mom. It would only be many years later that she would look back on those days and realize the gift she received from her mother. She received faith and strength her mother and those values would help Nora find her pathways forward in life. Frederick Douglass was not thinking of strong girls 150 years ago when he talked about building strong children, only boys and then men got such attention. But Nora would end up being one of those children—strong, resilient, not broken, and thankful to her mom and her dad for building it in to her during the hardest childhood loss she could ever have imagined.

Nora and her dad both lived in the survival window, we talked about earlier, after the woman they both loved passed away. But eventually they chose hope. The research has become clear that if children and teens understand the science of hope, they are in a much better place to be able to apply it to their lives—whether the challenges come from abuse, natural disaster, an illness, or the loss of a loved one. Teaching children to measure their own hope and to understand what they can do to raise it, produces power in their life. A child who understands hope is a child empowered to pursue their dreams.

The Children's Hope Scale

The Children's Hope Scale was published by Rick Snyder in 1997. Children who can identify pathways (waypower) toward their goals and exert agency (willpower) to sustain goal directed motivation are considered hopeful. The validated Children's Hope Scale is a six-item self-report of both pathways and agency thinking developed for children between the ages of 8 and 16. This scale uses three pathways and three willpower (agency) statements that can be added to generate a total Hope score. Like the Adult Hope Scale, higher total scores reflect higher hope among the child participants.

Researchers have consistently reported strong evidence for both validity and reliability of the Children's Hope Scale even in different languages. Validity means the results are accurate. Once you know these things, you can make a prediction. Rick Snyder could predict who would keep their hand in the cold water the longest on GMA based on the accuracy of the Adult Hope Scale. He knew Charlie Gibson's high Hope score would make him the winner on pain tolerance. Chan and others have proven the same thing with the Children's Hope Scale. It predicts long-term positive outcomes with children.

Can Young Children Really Answer the Hope Survey?

To our grandchildren, we are both Papa. We have special relationships with our grandchildren and we are obsessed with their level of hope. Every grandparent should be obsessed with the Hope scores of their grandchildren. The Children's Hope Scale is validated for ages 8 through 16. Chan has now conducted research that has helped demonstrate that even younger children can be confidently asked to complete the Children's Hope Scale. In the last four years, we have administered the Hope Scale to 6-8 year olds at Camp HOPE America and have found that even a 6-year-old can understand the concepts of the Hope Scale.

If you are an adult and don't work with children or have children, you can skip this section of the book. But for those that are teens or those that work with teens, the Children's Hope Scale should be an important tool in your journey. You can use this scale if you are a young person reading this book or you can reach out to us at info@ allianceforhope.com to receive a fillable version.

THE CHILDREN'S HOPE SCALE

Directions: Read each sentence carefully. For each sentence, please think about how you are in most situations. Using the scale shown below, please select the number that best describes YOU and put that number in the blank provided. There are no right or wrong answers.

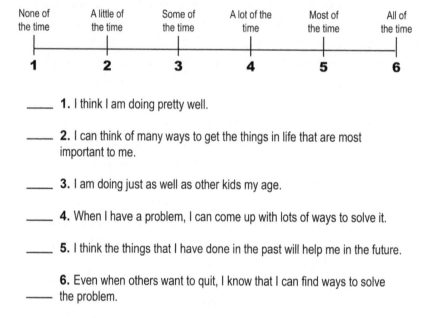

None of the time	A little of the time	Some of the time	A lot of the time	Most of the time	All of the time
1	**2**	**3**	**4**	**5**	**6**

_____ **1.** I think I am doing pretty well.

_____ **2.** I can think of many ways to get the things in life that are most important to me.

_____ **3.** I am doing just as well as other kids my age.

_____ **4.** When I have a problem, I can come up with lots of ways to solve it.

_____ **5.** I think the things that I have done in the past will help me in the future.

_____ **6.** Even when others want to quit, I know that I can find ways to solve the problem.

Notes: The **Agency** subscale score is the sum of items 1, 3 & 5; the **Pathways** subscale score is the sum of items 2, 4 & 6. **Hope** is the sum of the three **Pathways** and three **Agency** items. Scores can range from a low of 6 to a high of 36.

Agency Score   _____ (Add items 1,3 and 5)

Pathways Score   _____ (Add items 2,4, and 6)

Total Hope Score _____ (Agency Score + Pathways Score)

Understanding a Child's Hope Score—Hope in Action

The Children's Hope Scale has been administered to thousands of children in many programs. Scores of 30 or above put you in a high hope category. Scores below 30 demonstrate hope at a moderate level. Scores from 12-18 register hope but at low levels. Scores below 6 put a child or teen in a low hope category. What does it mean if a child is low in hope? It just means there is work to do. Higher rates of childhood adversity tend to reduce Hope scores in most human beings and this includes children. This makes our work with children more challenging but not impossible. Rising hope can blunt the impact of childhood trauma. Our guess is that the Hope score you find in some children and teens will not surprise you. But the good news again, is hope can rise. Using Rick Snyder's case scenario approach, let's look at three children from our camping and mentoring work that can tell us about Hope in Action in children with major trauma in their lives.

Jardon—A Hot Wind: High Willpower/Low Waypower
Jardon experienced violence in his home from his earliest memories. He doesn't remember much about his father but what he does remember is not good. The wind blew hot in the summer on the street he lived on as a young child in El Centro, CA. 115 degrees was not uncommon during the summer months. The apartment had an air conditioner but it seemed broken most of the time. Going outside into the blazing sun was no escape from the heat. He could not remember much about his father though he would later learn his dad was 6'2", toned, and strong. His dad too had grown up with an abusive father. His dad fathered children with three women. He was a serial monogamist. Jardon was from his dad's second wife. Jardon's dad left to find his third wife when Jardon was just 6 years old. Jardon grew up with anger as his mom self-medicated her way through his elementary school years with alcohol and then methamphetamines. At age 9, Child Protective Services removed him after he came to school with meth in his backpack. He had found it in his mom's underwear drawer. His first foster mother received more than $700 per month to house him. On his first night, she was kind as the CPS worker brought him into the home and stayed for an hour to talk as he got settled in a small room off the kitchen. There was nothing on the walls. A tiny window was too high to see out of and lighting was a stained drop ceiling with one functioning and one burned out fluorescent tube. Within days, his foster mom was clear: "You don't have any rights here. You will do what I say or I will whoop your ass." He did not do what she said and he paid the consequences. He was only 9 years old. It was not a fair fight.

Jardon traveled through six foster homes between 9 and 14 years old. Each time CPS would conclude that it was not a good fit or the foster parents would ask to return him. The rejection burned a deeper and deeper wound in his soul as Jardon grew into a young man. He was athletic like his Dad and the anger of his unmet expectations fueled him in sports. He was strong, fast, and driven. No one ever crossed him or they felt his rage instantly. But coaches and teachers also experienced his rage and it got him kicked off every sports team. School was never his strong suit. He didn't read at grade level and too much cortisol was pumping through his body too much of the time after spending years in abusive and unsupportive foster homes.

By the time Jardon reached the group home, the system had decided he could not live with a family. Three years in the group home did not help Jardon's view of the world. He lived both angry and depressed. Anger for Jardon was not about listlessness or isolation in a dark room. His anger was an emotional reaction to his pain from rejection. But sometimes anger turns inward and forms a simmering form of depression. Jardon lived in that hot darkness most of the time.

Jardon's group home managers decided to sign him up for Camp HOPE in 2016. Imperial County was beginning the program and officials were looking for children to attend who had been impacted by violence and abuse. In violation of every Camp HOPE America policy on screening and selecting campers, the eight boys (ages 12-17) in the group home were all told they were going to camp because the group home managers wanted the week off.

Jardon boarded the bus to camp with marijuana in his front left pocket. At the first stop, he and three other boys lit up behind the rest stop bathroom. One of the adult volunteers smelled the dope and quickly identified the violators. They were defiant. That night, the Camp HOPE team made the decision that Jardon was not going on to camp. He had already brought drugs on the bus, threatened to hurt other children, and refused to listen to any instruction or direction. Imperial County CPS was notified and told to come get Jardon the next morning.

Jardon was told he was not going to camp because of his choices. Jardon's rage exploded toward one of the Camp HOPE staffers within minutes. He pushed his way back into the room where all the male campers were getting their sleeping bags ready for the night, screamed epithets at the group, and then went outside—announcing that he was going to camp whether anyone liked it or not. The Sheriff's Department was called and soon deputies arrived. As soon as they appeared, Jardon pulled out a Bluetooth speaker, connected it to his phone and began blaring music on the grass outside the rooms where terrified campers tried to settle down for the night. As the deputies approached, Jardon held up his phone in one hand and his speaker in the other and advanced on the officers screaming "Black lives matter, black lives matter." It was a scene that has played itself out across America in a host of situations—a conflict with a black man ends up in officers opening fire. But the deputies kept it low and slow and quickly realized that Jardon did not have a gun. Jardon was briefly subdued and later released to a CPS worker who returned him to his group home. Jardon never went to Camp HOPE.

Jardon had expectations as a child. He wanted a father to love him. He wanted to be safe. He wanted to be happy. His expectations survived abuse, foster care, and the group home. Even in his anger and pain, he remained high in willpower. But Jardon had little waypower. The further he fell behind in school, without any help, the lower his waypower went. Athletics were his outlet for his rage, but his confrontations with coaches and teachers stigmatized him and destroyed options for his future. Jardon's journey is not over but professional mental health intervention is likely his only pathway forward toward hope until the criminal justice system claims him and designates his pathway to jail or prison.

Dalia—Hidden in a Hoodie: Low Will, High Ways

Dalia was born in Mexico. Her mom and dad separated when she was very young. Her mom remarried when she was 6. Dalia remembers crying on the day her mom re-married because her stepdad told her they would be moving to the United States. She knew the marriage would mean leaving her family, relatives, and friends. She barely knew her stepdad when he married her mother. Her stepdad was nice at first but soon the controlling and abusive behavior started. He was an alcoholic and verbally, emotionally, and physically abusive. Dalia lived constantly in fear and apprehension. Her mom finally left with Dalia and her siblings after six years of abuse. They were homeless and in and out of shelters for three years. They lived on food stamps and welfare. She remembers being sad most of the time—always feeling like things were missing from her life but not quite sure what. She made friends easily but changed schools often so nothing lasted.

Dalia came to Camp HOPE for the first time at age 13. She arrived hidden in a hoodie, with the drawstring pulled tight to hide her face. She was dark, withdrawn, and quiet. Her first Hope score was extremely low. In her words, "I was a messed-up kid with a f--- life attitude. I had no motivation to do anything. I didn't even know what hope was and when people talked about it I didn't care." The first few days she did not talk much or share her story. Her first pictures during art one day at camp caught everyone's attention. They were dark but stunning. Dalia was a gifted artist. As everyone praised her giftedness, Dalia's hoodie string slowly loosened. "You can be an artist, Dalia." "You can make money doing this." "You are so talented." As the first week of camp came to an end, the hoodie was off and Dalia even smiled from time to time—a beautiful, sad smile but, nevertheless, a smile. Hope rising.

The second year she attended camp it was obvious to all that a window had opened into Dalia's heart. She laughed and smiled when she got on the bus to go to camp. She was funny and more outgoing. The hoodie was gone and her beautiful face and flowing black hair revealed a girl who knew she was talented and capable. Dalia recorded a video for Camp HOPE America and shared how much she loved s'mores, rafting, hiking, and "talking about my feelings." School did not really excite her but she was finding herself in art and humor. Both art and humor were outlets for her pain and her anger towards her mom was beginning to fade. "I realized my mom did the best she could. She grew up with abuse too and when my mom finally told about her abuse as a child, no one believed her." Dalia said counseling started to help when she began to understand why she had the feelings she did and began to realize she could have goals in her life.

At age 17, Dalia began to think about forgiving her Dad for leaving and for what he had done to her mom. Her dad was living and working in Mexico so seeing him was difficult but she decided to reach out. Three years of Camp HOPE had challenged her to choose forgiveness as the best way to look forward toward hope in her life. She talked to her Dad on the phone, texted with him, and began to plan a visit. Her dad told her he wanted to get to know her and try to have a relationship. One weekend, Dalia's dad called to see if she could come down to Mexico. But she had plans and was not sure if she was fully ready. She told him they would get together soon. The next Tuesday, Dalia's dad was shot and killed by an unknown assailant. Dalia's world was devastated. The darkness she struggled with so many times in her younger years returned. Her regret and grief made it hard to breathe. Her dad was gone and she would never have a relationship with him, never resolve the deep hurt, never get to tell him she loved him. The darkness of that pain caused Dalia to think about taking her own life. It was a normal reaction to a terrible tragedy in her life.

Dalia came to Camp HOPE for the fourth year just two days after her dad's funeral. Her pain was raw. She was focused only on survival. But she had found a community of support at Camp HOPE and amidst the pain she said on the first day of camp, "I didn't want to come this week but I really need to be here with all of you." Throughout the week she talked about how paralyzing her dad's death was to her and how easy it would be to lose her motivation for school and her future. She talked about ending her life. She said the pain just made her want to somehow forget what had happened. She described the temptation to medicate or drink as her broken heart made her feel so sad. Dalia needed her friends and the Camp HOPE team to just hug her, love her, tell her how sorry everyone was, and encourage her to live her life to honor her dad's memory.

Dalia's story is not over. She is a senior in high school. She has pathways and the ability to find them. But her willpower, her motivation to move forward, is hampered by the pain and sadness she has experienced. She needs to focus on surrounding herself with friends that encourage her, adults that can support her, and father figures that believe in her. They are the best substitute for a father she will find right now.

Allan—Missing Out on Life: Low Will, Low Ways
Allan's dad hit his mom often. The violence started when she was pregnant with Allan. Allan doesn't have many positive memories of childhood except for being with his sister June. June is two years younger than Allan and often looked up to him as her big brother and he took on the role of her protector. His dad was gone by the time he was in 6th grade. It was for the best. The violence ended and Allan, June, and their mom tried to navigate life without the constant fear. Allan was a quiet boy with a love of science and math. Video games were often his escape from reality. He is smart but the journey through child abuse and domestic violence sucked much of his motivation and drive during his elementary and middle school years.

June and Allan came to Camp HOPE for the first time when June was 12 and Allan was 14. Their mom signed them up after starting counseling at the San Diego Family Justice Center. Neither one of them had ever been camping and didn't think they had any interest. Allan found out he had to give up his phone and his laptop for the week and snakes in his sleeping bag seemed like a better idea than no electronics! But they came to camp and slowly embraced adventure, adrenaline, and laughter. It was not as lonely as being home alone together as their mom worked two jobs to pay the bills. And camp was the first time that Allan started hearing about "college" and had people asking him the question "What do you want to be when you grow up?" His mom dropped out of high school and his dad never finished ninth grade so Allan did not give much thought to his future before Camp HOPE.

As Allan spent more time going to the year-round activities of Camp HOPE, for the first time he started thinking about his own dreams. He had never seen any way to a different life and had never really thought he could be someone that was special or important. June though made a bad choice, looking for love, when she was 15 and got pregnant with her boyfriend. He was mad at June but also understood how much she really wanted someone to love her. Allan realized that June was not setting goals in her life and pregnancy became her way to deal with her anger toward her dad and her inability to see her future.

As Allan learned more about college and learned more about how his own actions were connected to his lack of motivation, he began to realize that he could have dreams and goals. Yesenia Aceves, the Director of the Camp HOPE America year-round mentoring program in San Diego, challenged Allan to think about being a counselor for camp when he graduated from high school. Yesenia described her first impression of Allan this way: "He was very quiet and introverted and kept mostly to himself. When I talked to him, he would only give short answers, nod, and smile. But he was polite and kind and I thought he could be a good counselor for other children." Yesenia's belief in Allan caused him to say "Yes" to being a counselor though he later confided to others that he was "terrified" that he might let Camp HOPE down. Becoming a counselor for others helped Allan begin to think about his ability to support other children learning to navigate their way out of violence and abuse in their homes. In 2017, Allan became one of the first graduates of the year-round Pathways program and received a $1,500 Verizon Foundation stipend as he began college. Allan wants to be a psychologist and "help other kids like me."

Allan's willpower and his waypower have risen dramatically since age 14 and his Hope scores (completed each year at camp and twice during the year) confirm it. He started very low in hope and is now much higher. He has more challenges ahead of him and there will be obstacles and difficulties. But Allan called the Camp HOPE America office recently to confirm that he wanted to come back and be a counselor again. He is helping others and helping himself to ensure his hope level stays high as he navigates his way into adulthood.

The consequences of low hope are never good. Low hope produced the rage of Jardon and the hopelessness of Dalia after her Dad's death. But understanding the science of hope helped Dalia and Allan find the motivation and identify the pathways toward hope and healing. They needed cheerleaders in their lives to increase their motivation to set goals. They needed to realize they were having normal reactions to abnormal experiences so they could reject the shame and blame that so easily settled over them. But measuring hope and then increasing hope has mattered. Children like Allan and Dalia can point the way forward for all of us—conscious choices to creating rising hope no matter what we have experienced in the past.

Measuring and Increasing Hope in All Children

Hope should be measured in all children, not just trauma-exposed children. The earliest hope research with elementary, middle, and high school students was done by then-graduate students at the University of Kansas including Dr. Lisa Edwards, Dr. Alicia Ito, and Dr. Jennifer Teramoto Pedrotti in their work with Rick Snyder, Shane

Lopez and Tom Krieshock. It helped shape research now being done by Gallup with millions of students in schools across the country.

The earliest research is instructive and the findings are consistent with our work with abused children in Camp HOPE America. Nearly 20 years ago, in Kansas, the researchers created a program called Making Hope Happen (MHH) in a middle school. Every student in their study took the Children's Hope Scale at the beginning of the program. Some students were then placed in a control group and did not get to go through the MHH program. For those that did get to do the program, they attended five 45 minute sessions in groups of 8-10 middle schoolers. Each group of students was led by two graduate students. They explained the definition of hope to the students (goals, pathways, agency). In Week 1, using posters and cartoons, the graduate students helped the kids learn about hope including biographical characters that lived high hope lives and made statements about their goals and accomplishments that the kids could study. Each child was challenged to pick a personal goal—big or small. The goal did not have to be accomplished within five weeks but it needed to be a positive goal, versus a negative goal. "I want to stop fighting with my sister" was a negative goal. A positive goal for this could be "I want to have a better relationship with my sister." Then, each student was paired with a "Hope Buddy" to spend time together during the five-week program at times. They paired a high hope child with a low hope child in each buddy relationship with the goal of promoting modeling through the program for children with low hope. By week 2, they taught children an acronym—G-POWER. What did it stand for? G = goals; P = pathways; O = obstacles; W = willpower; E = evaluate your process; R = rethink and try again. They memorized the acronym. By Week 3, the children learned a board game called the "Hope Game" where they had to set goals, look for motivation, and figure out pathways to get to their game goals. By Week 4, the concept of "hope talk" was introduced.

With hope talk, students were asked to change unhopeful sentences to more hopeful. "I will never be good at math" could become "Math is not my best subject, but I can find strategies to do better." Statements about hope by historical figures were studied and evaluated for their level of hopefulness. The last piece of Week 4 was helping children start writing their personal hope story including talking about their original goal and the progress they had made toward the goal even if it wasn't accomplished yet. In the final week of the MHH Program, children read their hope stories to the group and there was a party to celebrate the progress that the students had made. What was the result?

Hope rising. Children going through the program had increased Hope scores compared to the control group. Later, the results were repeated in elementary schools and high schools. Across the board, it became clear that you can teach children the science of hope and then they can work the plan to increase their own Hope scores.

Later, graduate students at the University of Kansas created the "Hope Camera Project" to see if creative group efforts with photography could increase hope using the same five week program model with students. They gave each student a disposable camera with instructions to go take pictures of people, places, or things that represented hope to each of them. The program included biographical characters just like the other experiments and teaching on the elements of the science of hope from week to week. Over the weeks, each student also took pictures and then designed a final "Hope Project" with their own pictures. Some students made collages, some made Power Point presentations, others made a musical presentation. One student lost his disposable camera, borrowed a video camera and got the help of other students to make a movie instead of using still photos (pathways thinking!). In week 5, they all shared their projects with the other students, took their Hope scores again, measured them, and then had a party. What were the results?

You guessed it. Hope rising. Students had major increases in hope in five weeks. In every project, it became clear that children and teens can be taught the science of hope and then they can learn to increase it in their own lives. Students with low hope naturally had the largest increases in hope. Former Oklahoma Governor Brad Henry said it years ago this way, "A good teacher can inspire hope, ignite the imagination, and instill a love of learning." The school-based teaching about the science of hope confirmed everything Brad Henry espoused.

So, if this is so obvious, why isn't every school in America teaching hope? Why isn't every youth program focused on hope? We still have work to do. And hope is not just for kids. It is for women, men, and children of all ages. It is even for the elderly.

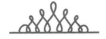

Chapter 7

Experiencing Hope

"Infuse your life with action. Don't wait for it to happen. Make it happen. Make your own future. Make your own hope. Make your own love. And whatever your beliefs, honor your creator, not by passively waiting for grace to come down from upon high, but by doing what you can to make grace happen... yourself, right now, right down here on Earth."

—Bradley Whitford

Colette

Colette's husband died at the age of 79. After 58 years of marriage, his sudden death from a heart attack was devastating. He was her best friend, the love of her life, and her caregiver as she struggled with the beginning signs of dementia. They had stayed the course—through four children, five jobs, great joys, deep sorrows, exciting adventures, cancer, retirement, and mental illness—in their commitment "until death do us part." Now, it was time for the death part. Though 81 years old, she had never lived on her own, never paid the bills, and never even planned a trip by herself. She was a mother and a grandmother, but her primary identity had been "wife" for her entire adult life. The goals she had with her husband were now gone. There would never again be a pathway for their goals. Her heartbreak was a deep pain that never went away. She had been diagnosed with dementia and every daily task was difficult for her. She was broken by her loneliness. Was there another chapter for her life? Was there any way she could go on? She told her children for months that she wished she could just die and go be with the man she loved.

Colette could no longer live alone so her children sold her home and moved her into an independent living apartment in a continuing care retirement community in San Diego called Mt. Miguel Covenant Village. She agreed she would try to learn to live on her own. But filled with fear and doubt, it was hard to imagine life without her soulmate. Nights were the worst. But mornings were not much better. She would lay in bed and wonder why she should get up. When your memories are more powerful than your dreams, life begins to end. Her memories were all she was hanging on to, day after day. Her new doctor diagnosed her with depression and then Parkinson's disease. The future of life on this earth was dark and hopeless.

The goals she started setting were small at first. Get out of bed. Get dressed. Say hello to one person every day. Ask someone a question about their life. Her children and grandchildren rallied around her. They visited often. They planned outings, family gatherings, and special times for her. Her goals grew. Decorate the apartment for Christmas. Bake a pie for a friend. Walk in the gardens. Pay the bills on her own. Buy a new car. Pass the driving test. Go to Hawaii. Hope began rising as she accomplished one goal and then another.

She started talking about her heartbreak. She agreed to fight the long goodbye of Parkinson's and dementia for as long as she could. She agreed, that when she was ready, she would open her heart to new friendships. She accepted the challenge to go to social events and try to meet new people. She promised she would trust God to help her find reasons why she was still alive even though her husband was gone. Her choice to have goals and her willingness to ask her children to help her find pathways forward helped her experience hope even in the most heartbreaking time of her entire life. She also knew that she could not do everything she wanted to do. She had always wanted to have her own art studio. There was no pathway. She would have to create a small area in her one bedroom apartment for her art. She drove for as long as she could and realized she no longer had the necessary focus to safely do this. She sold her car. She wanted to cook her own meals as well since she had cooked for her family throughout her life. She cooked for herself for nearly five more years. But she eventually realized she had to pick and choose where she focused her energy.

Colette fell in love again almost two years after her husband's death. She was 82 years old. Her "boyfriend" Jim was 92. They never married, but they loved each other for nearly six years. Her family hired a driver for them and they went on dates. They sat on her porch and held hands. She even confided to her son what a great kisser Jim was! They became inseparable. Scooter rides together were a highlight of many days after she lost the ability to walk. Colette went peacefully into eternity on March 17, 2016. Jim sat at her bedside and sang to her and held her hand until she was in the presence of her God.

Hope is not just for the young or for those with a long life ahead of them. There are millions of seniors in this country who need rising hope in their lives. Colette experienced the science of hope even if she never would have called it that. She found desired goals (living well on her own and making new friends), and chose pathways (going to social events and introducing herself). As she accomplished a goal, she began to experience hope. When she first began the pathway to a difficult goal of living well on her own, she experienced uncertainty, fear, and doubt. It was not a linear journey. She struggled with depression and loneliness at times. However, as she gained success (achieving steps toward her goal), her confidence (and self-efficacy) began to increase. In the early phase of her journey after her husband's death, her ability to dedicate *willpower* to the *pathway* was important especially as she experienced barriers that needed to be overcome.

Colette's family played a powerful role in cheering for her and motivating her. In the later part of her journey, she needed to deploy her willpower more selectively (depending on the goals she was pursuing at any given time). To complicate her experience, she faced attention detractors. That is, as she pursued her desired goal, she had to pay attention to the other domains of her life that demanded her mental energy and make choices.

This is true for all of us. In graduate school, Chan had goals he wanted to achieve, such as publishing his research. During law school, Casey had goals of exercising daily and traveling for fun and adventure. During this same time, however, we were both employed full-time (work domain), had a family that deserved our attention (family domain), and had to study for the courses we were taking (school domain). We had to make choices on what we prioritized and what we let fall by the wayside.

The key point is this: We pursue our goals in an environment that puts many demands on our time and energy. Competing demands can influence our capacity to hope. *It is not true that we can have it all.* We often need to choose between our goals and focus on those most important to us, and possibly defer some until a later time.

What are your attention detractors in your life right now? What is sucking your willpower and energy to prevent you from pursuing the goals you really have? Is it time to make a list of your most important goals and then take a few off so others can get your full attention? Colette kept some things on her list of goals and took others off. For years, she loved watching the news. But then it started to suck the life right out of her. She started saying, "The news puts me in a bad mood." News was

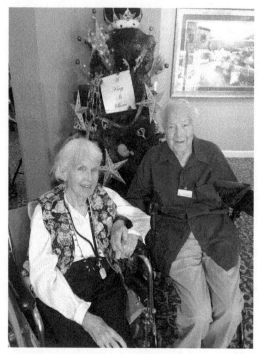

Colette with Jim (2016)

an attention detractor. The news was damaging her motivation to pursue her goals. She had to make a choice to turn it off so she could stay positive about her life.

Colette's high hope approach gave her eight amazing years at Mt. Miguel Covenant Village after her husband died. She made friends, fell in love with Jim, and lived independently until she passed into eternity at age 88. Colette's experience of hope should inspire all of us. She was Casey's mom and he got to see the science of hope up close and personal in her life.

We can all have high hope even amidst the greatest challenges of life. We just have to make the decision that we really want to experience it—not once, but over and over, day by day. You need to make hope happen. Truth: Hope is a verb.

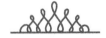

Chapter 8

The Hope Continuum

"Hope has two beautiful daughters; their names are Anger and Courage. Anger at the way things are, and Courage to see that they do not remain as they are."
—Augustine of Hippo

Laural

I stood next to my mom, securely attached to her leg as she hung out the clothes. I was two years old and later would tell a counselor it was my first memory in life. I recall a sense of comfort and safety in that moment. It was the last time I would have those feelings for many years. My father began molesting me when I was 3.

Raised in a middle-class family in Northern California, my upbringing was typical for a child of the 1950s. Gender roles were fixed and clear. Women were expected to be subservient to men. In elementary school, I beat a boy in a race and excitedly told my mother that I was the fastest person in my school. My mom responded, "Laural, you have to let him win because he is a boy." The message was clear: Men and boys are in charge and girls and women must remember that in every situation. My parents divorced when I was 8 years old.

I vividly recall mornings after the divorce, when my father would take me to his bed. The furniture, the ceiling light, his smell, his behavior, asking if I liked this or that, were all part of the scene in my mind. I learned to dissociate and leave my body while it was happening. But afterwards, I was not dissociated. I remember my dad taking me into the shower and washing off my genitals. "Don't tell your mother about this because she wouldn't like it." No one knew about the sexual abuse and I never told but my anger was deep.

By the time I left home and began dating, I had learned a lesson. My job was to give men sexual satisfaction. Predators quickly found me and I was sexually assaulted hundreds of times. My predators would view my acquiescence as consent. I eventually fell in love and married a man who did not use or abuse me. But by then my patterns of behavior were deeply entrenched in my life. I continued to be sexually involved with men whenever they made any effort to use me for their sexual gratification. By age 40, I saw no pathways except suicide or counseling. I decided to try counseling.

My male counselor gained my trust, learning my vulnerabilities and triggers. And then he sexually abused me. I was broken, devastated, and deep in the darkness of despair.

Months later, I decided to try a female counselor and found support, care, and a pathway forward in life. It took years to rebuild my marriage and let go of my shame and self-loathing. I sued my former therapist and won. I started setting goals around my life, my marriage, and my family. I found ways to help other abused children and share my story with others who had lived my nightmare—helping them find hope and healing.

Laural lived what we call the Hope Continuum.

The Hope Continuum

What is the opposite of hope? When we ask this question, the most common response we receive is hopelessness. But hopelessness is not quite the opposite of hope. To better understand the loss of hope, ask yourself, what is hopelessness? Hopelessness occurs when the outcome is already determined and there is nothing you can do to change it from happening. The result is reflective of singer John Cougar's album title, "Nothing Matters and What If It Did?" Hopelessness looks a little different than we might think.

Those who have experienced repeated failures when attempting to achieve their goals are unlikely to understand they lack pathways and/or willpower, nor would they articulate the problem in that way. But repeated failure at goal attempts often results in reduced hope. As hope declines, individuals will react to goals with a focus

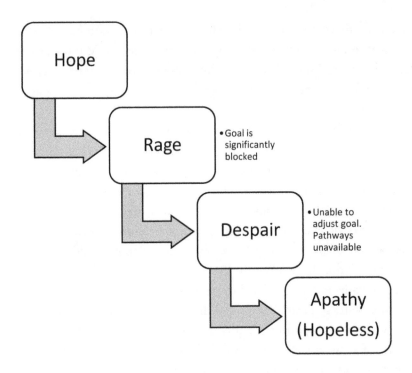

on failure and negativity such as anger, frustration, or sadness. The graphic below explains the spectrum that most experience when hope is reduced.

Phase I (Anger/Rage): When we cannot achieve our desired goals, we tend to react with anger, frustration, or rage. Laural lived with the rage of what happened to her throughout her childhood. In adulthood, the rage lived on even as she used it to motivate her at times.

Anger and rage are the closest emotions to hope. Anger is not bad, rage is not wrong. *To put it simply, anger, frustration, and even rage are NORMAL responses when our expectations do not meet our lived experience.* Anger is not the enemy. What we do with our rage and anger is the issue, not whether we feel the frustration of blocked goals. Laural's anger was a natural reaction to an abnormal situation she was experiencing. Fathers are not supposed to molest their children. Laural wanted comfort and safety from her parents, just like every child does. When her goal was not reality, it produced anger.

Black Lives Matter
One great example of the relationship between hope and anger is Black Lives Matter (BLM). BLM has generated both enormous support and strong criticism. It is an

international activist movement in the African-American community that campaigns against violence and systemic racism towards black people. BLM often protests police killings and broader issues of racial profiling, police brutality, and racial inequality. BLM began after George Zimmerman was acquitted for killing Trayvon Martin in Florida in 2013.

BLM is an organization motivated by the anger that comes when expectations and goals cannot be achieved. Our first African-American President, Barack Obama, could not solve hundreds of years of racial oppression and discrimination. Though Barack Obama ran on a "Hope" platform, there was no way that one man could produce goals and pathways to address every racial issue in America for everyone who had experienced violence, historic oppression, and injustice. George Zimmerman's acquittal became a flashpoint, much like Ferguson, Missouri would produce yet again in 2014 when Officer Darrin Wilson shot and killed Michael Brown.

Barack Obama never articulated the science of hope but he became the President of the United States by raising the hope of the American public. No one ever measured the hope of people supporting Obama, but if it had been measured before he was elected and after he was elected we would have seen rising hope. President Obama set goals and convinced millions of Americans that there were pathways to those goals. He painted a picture of the future that people believed could become a reality. President Obama proved the words of Napoleon Bonaparte true, "A leader is a dealer in hope."

BLM is, in many ways, the natural frustration that comes for many that believed in his goals and his pathways. Not all his goals were achieved. The natural outcome is anger, particularly given the many obstacles that opponents and those with other views put in his way. And the anger was latent before Barack Obama's run for President. Decades and decades of oppression played a role in producing seething anger toward injustice and racism only exacerbated by the deaths of George Floyd and many others.

Interestingly, President Donald Trump articulated a very different set of goals and pathways for America. Yet those who voted for him embraced his vision of the future and likely experienced higher hope because of their belief that Donald Trump could produce the America they wanted. Hope is amoral. Goals and pathways can be about better financed government-funded health care or they can be about less government regulation of health care. Trump voters loved his goals for less immigration, less military support for other countries, a big wall on the southern border, and lower taxes. "America first" was a very different goal than anything that Barack Obama articulated. But the science is the same. For BLM, anger was the result when goals were not achieved because pathways were not available. This was the result for Trump as well, as his supporters saw that goals were not achieved and pathways did not exist for everything he promised. The Capitol riot on January 6, 2021 was the rage of Trump supporters about goals not achievable.

An abused child experiences rage in much the same way that BLM has at a societal level. We just looked at Laural's internalized rage. Children long to have parents who love and care for them. Those expectations are destroyed when violence and abuse is unleashed on a child or on a child's mother by her father. The result: Rage. Expectations are different than lived experience. Goals do not have pathways. We will come back to the challenges of turning rage into hope later, but understanding how close rage is to hope is a central part of the science we will come to appreciate in this book.

Phase 2 (Despair): The second phase of reduced hope is despair. This occurs when viable alternatives are not available (pathways) or we cannot adjust our goal. In this condition, the barriers appear insurmountable. Laural got there in her journey. She had goals all the way into marriage with her husband, but those goals to have a healthy, honest, faithful relationship had no pathways given her major trauma from childhood and her inability to stop engaging other men sexually. With despair, the goal remains desirable, but there is a pathways or agency problem. The individual is experiencing the loss of hope but is not yet hopeless as they continue to direct mental energy (agency) toward the object of their desire. We saw Dalia's despair just after her dad died. Laural lived the same experience of despair.

Tens of thousands of Americans working in dead end jobs or unhealthy work environments today experience Phase 2 in the loss of hope. Anger eventually turns into despair when people cannot find a way to adjust their employment goals or find a pathway to improve their work environments. The result is discouragement, sometimes numbness, and the slow bleed of hope from our lives. If you are living with low hope in your work environment, you feel the truth of the research. If you have a high hope work environment, try asking a few friends and neighbors about their work environment. Try a few of these questions: What are your goals at work right now? Do you have pathways to achieve those goals? Who is cheering for you at work, helping to motivate you to achieve your goals? It will quickly become clear if they are low hope or high hope about their work. If they are experiencing despair, loss of motivation, no pathways or blocked goals, it will become obvious very quickly.

Phase 3 (Apathy): The final phase in the loss of hope is apathy. The goal is not possible *and* no mental energy (agency) is expended either toward the goal or searching for pathways that may lead to the goal. Apathy is the opposite of hope as it refers to the absence of motivation and goal focused energy. Many of us know someone who ends up apathetic—a student, a friend, a co-worker, or a family member. It presents itself as "I don't give a shit anymore" or "I give up."

Consider the example of a middle-school child who lays their head on the desk at school and is not engaged in learning. When the teacher attempts to prod the child into the lesson, the child responds with a focus on failure ("I can't do it") or negativity expressed as anger toward the teacher or others. In rage, the child might express it this way: "I don't care anymore" or "I don't give a shit." The teacher's typical response to this scenario is to send the child to detention or suspension—trying to discipline them or punish the inappropriate language or behavior. Anyone working with the child who does not understand the science, might shame or blame the child. But what is happening in this moment is the result of low hope. There is a better response, informed by our new understanding. A trauma-informed, hope-centered teacher will patiently, carefully, lovingly meet the child where he or she is and focus on what is behind those low hope statements, not focus on the offensive language that is only symptomatic of the real issues.

What we offer with the science of hope is an important alternative to the typical response of a teacher or authority figure. In the example above, the child is apathetic in the classroom. Apathy is the opposite of hope so we must consider both pathways and agency solutions. The apathetic child does not see the classroom or education as a pathway toward desirable goals. Most likely there is also trauma in the child's life that has played into a low Hope score. Making the time to hear about the child's fears, frustrations, and trauma, should be part of the solution. While it is easy to oversimplify this scenario, spending time trying to understand, identify, or inspire even a small goal with an apathetic child may allow for a connection where the classroom can become a potential pathway to that goal. This careful, thoughtful nurturing of hope in an apathetic child by a teacher and/or parent can change the trajectory of the child's life if done in a thoughtful, hope-centered way. Our research shows that rising hope can become a protective factor in the lives of apathetic children and adults and can change the destinies of many living at the opposite end of the spectrum from hope.

One other point is important in understanding the Hope Continuum. Children or adults can be moving down the Continuum and still take each level of emotion with them. Rage may remain even as despair sets in. Rage and despair may travel with apathy even when a child or adult sees no way forward in life. The stages of hope are not mutually exclusive.

Laural found hope out of the worst imaginable child abuse and related rage. Colette, brokenhearted by the death of her husband of 58 years, eventually found her way out of despair and apathy to hope. Did you have experiences in childhood that robbed you of hope? Have you experienced the anger of unfulfilled expectations in your life that that leaves you emotionally separated from hope? If you are not high in hope now right now, were you once? What happened to steal it? Many of us—nearly 70% of the American public—have experiences from childhood that negatively impact our natural bent toward high hope. But we can regain it as well. Most of this book is focused on how we do that. But first let's understand it from the most significant study ever done on the predictive impact of childhood experiences on our level of hope in both childhood and later in life. It may shed light on why so many of us struggle to make hope real in our lives.

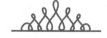

Chapter 9

The Adverse Childhood Experiences (ACE) Study

"Teach the children so it will not be necessary to teach the adults."
—Abraham Lincoln

Christian

The fire crackled. The light was fading. The darkness was being held at bay by the glow of the flames. Children faced the fire, sitting on logs, and listened intently to the question posed from Michael Burke, one of our camp leaders. "Where did you see hope today?" Hands shot up around the campfire circle. The first child, waved his arm, drawing Michael's attention. "I saw hope today when Allie was too scared to get in the boat. She was standing there but didn't want to get in but then she did. Everyone was cheering and yelling and she got in." "Way to go, Allie," Michael responded and everyone clapped. It was repeated ten or twelve times that night as it is every night at Camp HOPE. Then, I (Casey) stood up and talked to the kids about pursuing their dreams and choosing the future over the past. I shared part of my own story of abuse and then helped more than 50 children think about their dreams for the future. As the campfire burned down, kids began heading back to their tents, looking forward to rafting the next day on the Klamath River in Southern Oregon.

A 16-year-old named Christian asked me if he could talk to me instead of heading to his tent with his counselors and tent mates. "I need to tell you something," Christian paused. "You can talk to me, Christian," I offered softly. As we sat by glowing embers of the fire, Christian disclosed his truth. "I am going to kill myself on my 17th birthday." I knew we were on sacred ground. "Christian, how are you going to kill yourself?" "My parents have a braided rug in their garage. I am going to rap myself in it and then lay in the middle of the road below the crest of the hill near our house where the delivery trucks come into town late at night. There are no street lights. A truck will run over me." This was not just a suicidal idea. There was a plan. "Christian, have you written a suicide note?" "Yes. It is in the bottom of my mom's underwear drawer." I needed to be very careful with Christian.

"Do you have any other options besides killing yourself, Christian?" "No. I just don't care anymore. I can't change anything in my family. My dad will never change." "Christian, have you thought about moving out of your house?" "Yes, but I don't want to abandon my mom and brother." "But, Christian, you are going to abandon them when you kill yourself." For nearly twenty minutes, the conversation continued as the fire died out and everyone settled into their sleeping bags. Christian described his abusive father. He recounted how he had tried to do an "intervention" with his dad when he came home from work one day and his dad laughed at him and went to get a drink. The abuse had been going on for as long as Christian could remember. I challenged him to move out and promised to help him find a place he could go. "How about if you save yourself and then you can help your mom and brother?" It was a different goal and pathway than suicide.

Christian did move out and lived with a friend for a time to get away from his dad. He survived his 17th birthday. Within a year, his mom sought services at the Shasta County Family Justice Center. Christian worked full-time for Camp HOPE America the following summer and began to feel the impact of a rising Hope score. Today, Christian is a Junior at UCLA. He is majoring in neuroscience and wants to be a doctor. He has given a TED talk about his journey and has worked in a variety of programs with abused children. Christian is one of the hope heroes we celebrate in this book. His challenges are not gone. His journey is not linear. But he can articulate his goals and identify his pathways. His motivation comes from helping others and becoming a role model for his brother.

Christian's childhood trauma and abuse gave him an opportunity to find hope—goals and pathways—to a different life than he ever could have imagined that night by the campfire on the Klamath River. But tens of thousands of children and adults impacted by violence and abuse in their homes don't navigate out of their trauma. Their trauma damages their hope and often cuts their life short, destroys them, or turns them into predators or prey.

We define hope at Camp HOPE America as "believing in yourself, believing in others, and believing in your dreams" and then we help them see it, be it, and aspire to it. But childhood trauma is one of the greatest attackers of hope that many will ever face. It is important that we all understand its toxic impact before we embrace hope as the antidote.

In late 1999, Dr. Vincent Felitti came to a meeting of the San Diego Domestic Violence Council in San Diego. He was the Director of Preventative Medicine at Kaiser Permanente. He wanted to share findings from a study he was doing with the Centers for Disease Control and Prevention (CDC) in Atlanta connected with an obesity clinic he was running in San Diego for Kaiser Permanente. The room was filled with cops, prosecutors, advocates, therapists, probation officers, judges, and others working to help reduce domestic violence and related child abuse in San Diego. He presented his findings to everyone for 20 minutes about the "Adverse Childhood Experiences Study" and the relationship between childhood trauma and morbid obesity. No one got it. Then, the meeting went on as the group talked about things that really mattered to everyone.

Other topics that day in San Diego included how long batterers intervention programs should be for court-ordered abusers, the status of the local law enforcement investigations protocol on how to investigate domestic violence cases, and an upcoming fundraising event. Dr. Felitti's presentation was interesting but no one understood how it related to everyone's day to day work with victims of domestic violence and sexual assault.

At nearly the same time in Oklahoma, Dr. Chan Hellman was wondering how to measure success in stopping domestic violence and sexual assault and helping victims and their children. Early research on the science of hope was just beginning as well in the late 1990's with Rick Snyder's work at the University of Kansas, but no one was totally sure what it meant or how to define and measure it. No one was connecting childhood trauma with hope yet.

Today, our views have totally changed about the concept of hope and its relationship to childhood trauma. Our knowledge base has expanded dramatically. There is no doubt about the importance of the Adverse Childhood Experiences Study (ACE). The ACE study is the most significant piece of research ever done on the predictive nature of childhood trauma on adult illness, disease, criminality, and victimization.

There is strong evidence today that traumatic stress in childhood is closely related to the leading causes of morbidity, mortality, and disability in the United States: Cardiovascular disease, chronic lung disease, chronic liver disease, cancer, depression and other forms of mental illness, obesity, smoking, and alcohol and drug abuse. There is equally strong evidence that exposure to violence and abuse causes profound cognitive impacts and damages brain development. Children with severe exposure to violence and abuse are at much greater risk for PTSD, additional victimization, unhealthy and early sexual behaviors, delinquency, recruitment into human trafficking, and rage-based violence and abuse against others. The ACE Study and a great deal of other research has confirmed these realities.

A growing body of research has also established that rising hope reduces the impact of ACEs. Hope can counteract the destructive power of childhood trauma. Those with higher hope deal better with trauma than those with lower hope. The long-term impacts of ACEs are lessened when hope is higher.

Before we talk more about how to increase hope and apply the science to our lives, families, and our organizations, we must ALL be able to articulate the findings of the ACE Study. As we travel the country, we continue to be amazed at how few people know of the ACE Study and its implications. ACEs are a public health epidemic in this country, yet they are largely ignored in programs, policies, agencies, and even in the personal lives of those who are suffering the consequences of unmitigated trauma.

The Adverse Childhood Experiences Study

Dr. Vince Felitti and a team from Kaiser Permanente began work in the 1980's working with morbidly obese women and men in San Diego. Dr. Felitti was one of the leading preventive medicine experts in California at the time. He was focused on developing successful weight loss programs for extremely overweight women and men. The weight loss program used "supplemented fasting" which allowed participants to lose up to 300 pounds in a year without surgery. The program was extremely successful in helping people to lose large amounts of weight but had a high dropout rate after they were successful. Successful program graduates would become suicidal after losing 300 pounds. Others would turn to alcohol or drugs after graduation. One women regained 37 pounds in three weeks after successfully losing 300 pounds in less than a year without surgery. Others dropped out even after finding great success. Dr. Felitti began exploring the reasons for the high dropout rate and self-destructive behavior. He found a strong correlation between child sexual abuse and morbid obesity. Extreme obesity was sexually, physically, and emotionally protective for survivors of child sexual trauma and when women lost the weight they felt vulnerable again to potential abuse. Without obesity, they looked to find other "solutions" to their problems. They needed other coping mechanisms to dull the pain of what they had been through so many years ago.

Dr. Felitti later wrote: *"It became evident that traumatic life experiences during childhood and adolescence were far more common than generally recognized, were complexly interrelated and were associated decades later in a strong and proportionate manner with outcomes important to medical practice, public health, and the social fabric of a nation. In the context of everyday medical practice, we came to recognize that the earliest years of infancy and childhood are not lost, but like a child's footprints in wet cement, are often lifelong."*

Dr. Felitti's groundbreaking work around obesity and childhood trauma eventually led to the famous ACE Study. The ACE Study was conducted with Kaiser Permanente patients in cooperation with the CDC and eventually published by Dr. Felitti and Dr. Robert Anda from the CDC. Once the relationship between obesity and child sexual abuse became apparent, the next question was: What other types of childhood trauma might also have profound impacts on human beings over a long period of time? Felitti and Anda came up with a ten-question index of items to evaluate. Felitti needed only the support of Kaiser and their patients to find out what else might matter—things that happen to many of us before the age of 18.

The ACE study involved 17,421 Kaiser Permanente patients between 1995 and 1997 who agreed to share their life history. Participants were then followed for more than fifteen years. "Everything we've published comes from that baseline survey of 17,421 people," says Anda, "as well as what was learned by following those people for so long."

The ACE Questionnaire has become a validated instrument used in child welfare programs and many other settings. The ACE Study, which is nearing its 20th year, has found that children facing adversity from abuse or other forms of trauma do not fare well through childhood or later in life without intervention or other mitigating events in their life. Dr. Felitti is one of our personal mentors and his visionary work will have a profound impact for generations to come on those working with trauma-exposed children and adults.

The short- and long-term outcomes of these adverse child experiences include a multitude of health and social problems. The evidence is overwhelming and indisputable.

The ACE Questionnaire includes ten types of childhood trauma. Respondents mark each one they experienced before the age of 18. This produces a score between 0-10. The ACE score is then used to assess the total amount of traumatic stress during childhood. The ACE Study has demonstrated that as the number of ACEs increase, the risk for the following health problems increases in a strong and graded fashion:

- Alcoholism and alcohol abuse
- Chronic obstructive pulmonary disease (COPD)
- Depression
- Fetal death
- Health-related quality of life
- Illicit drug use
- Ischemic heart disease (IHD)
- Liver disease
- Risk for intimate partner violence
- Multiple sexual partners
- Sexually transmitted diseases (STDs)
- Smoking
- Suicide attempts
- Unintended pregnancies
- Early initiation of smoking
- Early initiation of sexual activity
- Adolescent pregnancy

The adverse childhood experiences that participants identified in the original ACE Study by Kaiser Permanente were categorized as Abuse, Neglect, and Household Dysfunction. The following subcategories were then assigned to each category:

Abuse
Emotional Abuse – Often or very often a parent or other adult in the household swore at you, insulted you, or put you down and sometimes, often or very often acted in a way that made you think that you might be physically hurt.

Physical Abuse—Sometimes, often, or very often pushed, grabbed, slapped, or had something thrown at you or ever hit you so hard that you had marks or were injured.

Sexual Abuse—An adult or person at least 5 years older ever touched or fondled you in a sexual way, or had you touch their body in a sexual way, or attempted oral, anal, or vaginal intercourse with you or actually had oral, anal, or vaginal intercourse with you.

Neglect

Emotional Neglect—Family members made you feel unloved and you did not feel special or important. Your family did not look out for each other or support each other.

Physical Neglect—Family members did not care for your physical needs, you did not have enough to eat, you wore dirty clothes, or no one took you to a doctor when you were sick.

Household Dysfunction

Mother Treated Violently—Your mother or stepmother was sometimes, often, or very often pushed, grabbed, slapped, or had something thrown at her and/or sometimes often, or very often kicked, bitten, hit with a fist, or hit with something hard, or ever repeatedly hit over at least a few minutes or ever threatened or hurt by a knife or gun.

Household Substance Abuse—You lived with someone who was a problem drinker or alcoholic or lived with anyone who used street drugs.

Household Mental Illness—A household member was depressed or mentally ill or a household member attempted suicide.

Parental Separation or Divorce—Parents were ever separated or divorced.

Incarcerated Household Member—A household member went to prison.

Higher ACE scores have now been correlated with drug and alcohol addiction, illness, disease, other destructive choices later in life, and reduced life expectancy. An ACE score of 6, for example, reduces life expectancy by nearly 20 years! Child trauma and adverse childhood experiences, without mitigating interventions and therapeutic help, are literally a pre-mature death sentence for many children exposed to violence, abuse, and trauma.

Not everyone in the ACE Study had high scores. Approximately one-third of the population (33%) in the study had an ACE score of 0. But more than 2/3 (67%) of the study participants had an ACE score of 1 or higher. If they had an ACE score of 1, 87% of those participants had at least one more trauma marker. This showed that people who had an alcoholic father, for example, were likely to have also experienced physical or verbal abuse. In other words, ACEs usually didn't happen in isolation. 1 in 6 individuals had an ACE score of 4 or more (12.4%). 1 in 9 individuals had an ACE score of 5 or more. Typically, the doctors and nurses found that the higher the ACE score the more difficult the patient was to deal with in a medical setting. Interestingly, women were 50% more likely than men to have an ACE score of 5 or more. 54% of depression and 58% of suicide attempts in women were attributed to adverse childhood experiences. Women of color scored even higher. High ACE scores also connected to other major negative consequences in the lives of trauma victims.

If you would like to evaluate your own ACE score, you can do it easily either right here in this book or online at www.hopescore.org, our website connected to this book. On our site, you can measure your Hope score and your ACE score.

We recommend every reader of the book find out their ACE score. The ACE Study confirms the old Biblical adage that "the sins of the parents are visited on the children to the third and fourth generations." This is not an academic exercise for either of us in writing this book. We too are children of ACEs. Chan has a score of 8 and Casey has a score of 5 on the ACE Scale. There is no shame in knowing your ACE score. It is the beginning of understanding your need for the power of rising hope in your life.

Below is the ACE Questionnaire if you want to take it before reading the rest of this book. Whether you aspire to be a mentor to other children, you are reading this book to process your own journey with trauma, or you want to be a better parent, it might be helpful to know your score. If you are a zero on the ACE Scale, you are blessed. It does not mean you don't have problems. It just means your problems are caused by other issues. But it will educate you on the impact of trauma in the lives of nearly 70% of those you know!

Any individual or group can use the ACE score sheet, but strong consideration should be given to providing emotional and psychological support for those completing the questionnaire in the event there is a score greater than zero. It can trigger significant trauma for participants, particularly those who have suffered sexual abuse.

We recommend that you talk to a close friend or de-brief with someone after calculating your ACE score, particularly if it is greater than zero.

The good news is that whatever your ACE score, you can overcome what happened to you as a child. But knowing the significance of an ACE score and what others around you with high ACE scores may face is important.

Over the years, the research confirms dramatically increased rates of drug and alcohol abuse, gang membership, generational abuse of children, violence against women, sexual victimization, and low levels of academic achievement in high ACE score children and teens. Christian struggled with these same kinds of impacts and even with rising hope in his life he may yet struggle more. The journey, as we have seen, is never linear.

Finding Your Own ACE Score

While you were growing up, during your first 18 years of life:

1. Did a parent or other adult in the household often or very often...
Swear at you, insult you put you down, or humiliate you?
OR Act in a way that made you afraid that you might be physically hurt?
Yes No If yes enter 1 _____

2. Did a parent or other adult in the household often or very often...
Push, grab, slap, or throw something at you?
OR Ever hit you so hard that you had marks or were injured?
Yes No If yes enter 1 _____

3. Did an adult or person at least five years older than you ever...
Touch or fondle you or have you touch their body in a sexual way?
OR Attempt or actually have oral, anal, or vaginal intercourse with you?
Yes No If yes enter 1 _____

4. Did you often or very often feel that...
No one in your family loved you or thought you were important or special?
OR Your family didn't look out for each other, feel close to each other, or support each other?
Yes No If yes enter 1 _____

5. Did you often or very often feel that...
You didn't have enough to eat, had to wear dirty clothes, and had no one to protect you? **OR** Your parents were too drunk or high to take care of you or take you to the doctor if you needed it?
Yes No If yes enter 1 _____

6. Were your parents ever separated or divorced?
Yes No If yes enter 1 _____

7. Was your mother or stepmother: Often or very often pushed, grabbed, slapped, or had something thrown at her? **OR**
Sometimes, often, or very often kicked, bitten, hit with a fist, or hit with something hard? **OR**
Ever repeatedly hit for at least a few minutes or threatened with a gun or knife?
Yes No If yes enter 1 _____

8. Did you live with anyone who was a problem drinker or alcoholic or who used street drugs?
Yes No If yes enter 1 _____

9. Was a household member depressed or mentally ill, or did a household member attempt suicide?
Yes No If yes enter 1 _____

10. Did a household member go to prison?
Yes No If yes enter 1 _____

Now, add up your "Yes" answers. This is your ACE score.

The correlations between ACEs and struggles later in life continue to be clear in research across the country. The higher the ACE score the more likely adults are to experience a host of negative consequences.

If your ACE score is 4, here are a few of the correlations that Dr. Felitti and others have identified in published studies referenced in the back of the book:

- 3600% more likely to become an injection drug (heroin) user (4600% at ACE of 6)
- 1200% greater likelihood of attempting suicide as an adult (2900% at ACE of 6)
- 1200% more likely to be a sexual assault victim
- 1000% more likely to inject street drugs
- 700% more likely to become an alcoholic
- 600% more likely to have sex before age 15
- 500% more likely to have multiple marriages
- 400% greater likelihood of emphysema or chronic bronchitis
- 390% more likely to have chronic obstructive pulmonary disease
- 300% more likely to contract HIV
- 300% more likely to become a domestic violence victim (woman); 150% (men)
- 300% greater likelihood of struggling with chronic depression
- 240% greater risk of hepatitis
- 240% higher risk of a sexually transmitted disease
- 200% more likely to become smokers
- 200% greater likelihood of severe obesity
- 150% more likely to have heart disease
- 100% greater risk of suffering from an auto-immune disease with ACE Score of 2>
- 51% of those with ACE Score of 4 will have behavioral problems in school (3% with ACE Score of 0)

When the ACE score is higher than 4, the likelihood of the behaviors above increases exponentially. Scores below 4 tend to reduce the likelihoods but do not eliminate these impacts unless the ACE score is zero. We don't include these to demoralize you or hinder hope in your life. Likelihoods and increased risk are not destinies. Many high ACE score human beings defy these odds and overcome the impacts of their childhood trauma. High hope weakens the impact of a high ACE score. We both have ACE scores higher than 4 and we have avoided most (though not all) of these impacts. But knowing them and being able to talk about them with each other has been cathartic and part of our healing. Your ACE score need not come with a huge dose of blame or shame. It does not have to be a dirty little secret that no one mentions. For many, understanding ACEs helps people feel normal. Your reactions to trauma in your life are normal reactions to abnormal experiences. You are not alone and you are not an anomaly. You likely have reacted to trauma the way most of us have even if you didn't understand why you made the choices you did.

We do believe strongly, however, that being able to talk about the trauma that you experienced as a child is crucial to long-term health. Talking and physical activity that releases trauma from the body are both possible—and they both relate to the science of hope. But the first piece must be honesty and transparency. A number of years ago a major researcher in this work took his own life and there has been no public discussion about it. His story of childhood trauma has never been told publicly. Too often our inability to talk about childhood trauma prevents us from being able to deal with it and release the pain from our minds and bodies. We will talk more about this later in the book when we talk about suicidal ideation, suicide, and murder-suicide.

ACEs should be part of every public health conversation in this country. Today, opioids are killing thousands but there is little conversation about the relationship to childhood trauma. More than 200,000 people have died from opioid use and abuse in the last 16 years and the connection to childhood trauma is clear from the ACE Study. Did you see it in our statistics above? If you are a 6 on the ACE Scale, the likelihood of using opioids goes up 4,600%. Dr. Robert Anda has said that this is the greatest correlation that most epidemiologists will see in their entire careers. Yet, there is scant discussion about it in the public health conversation about opioid use in the United States. In many cases, childhood trauma survivors, like child sexual abuse survivors in the original ACE Study, have found a solution to their pain. For child sexual abuse survivors, it was obesity. For others, it is heroin or some other version of opioids.

But there are other kinds of ACE stories. Parents who don't recognize them will miss the needs of their children after violence, trauma, or abuse.

Katie

In 2017, we both spoke at the International Family Justice Center Conference in Milwaukee, Wisconsin. We spent time with a beautiful 33-year-old woman named Katie. Katie was kidnapped from her home in Lodi, California when she was 12 years old and raped repeatedly. Her kidnapper was a rage-filled 25-year-old man named

Steven Cochran. She and her family did not know him. It was a crime of opportunity. He was watching the neighborhood and saw her parents leave for the evening. He then knocked on the door and asked for a phone book. Katie left to find one and returned to find him inside the front door of her home. Once inside the home, he assaulted both Katie and her sister though only Katie suffered actual sexual intercourse with Cochran. He then dragged Katie naked from the house—leading to a massive manhunt by San Joaquin County law enforcement over the next 20 hours. Katie was eventually found, having been assaulted multiple times, covered in mud, wandering in a field just a few miles from her house. The local news station described her as "muddy but safe." Another TV station called her "unharmed." Cochran was arrested, prosecuted, and is serving a life sentence. Katie was returned to her parents. They were given referrals for counseling and support. She went to counseling a few times but didn't want to keep attending. Katie was once again "safe" with her family and her parents saw little need to keep "bringing up" the trauma she had suffered.

But the consequences of Katie's traumatic and violent assault were not so easily addressed and she was not "unharmed." Her parents supported the counseling for a couple months and then wanted her life to go back to normal. She was OK. She was back with her sister and loving parents. Her parents did not encourage her to talk about it anymore. Katie did not even talk about it with her sister who had also been victimized.

Katie's trauma played itself out for years after the event. She started using drugs and alcohol in high school as she self-medicated her pain. She ended up in a series of abusive relationships as predators found this now sexually aware and traumatized young teenager. For 20 years Katie lived out the correlations of the ACE Study before finally hearing Casey present on it and realizing her reactions were normal. In the absence of trauma mitigation and high hope, Katie experienced normal reactions and consequences to an abnormal experience. But until she understood it, the effects were devastating.

Today, Katie has higher hope and cheerleaders in her life. She is finally finishing college and pursuing her dreams. Trauma almost destroyed her and rising hope finally gave her a way forward. She is very articulate now in saying how much she needed someone to tell her about the ACE Study and someone to help her understand the science of hope. We didn't understand the science twenty years ago when Katie was kidnapped but we do today. Now, we have no excuse when those around us need to understand the destructive nature of unmitigated trauma in their lives.

Katie was an inspiration to both of us. She needed far more help and information than she got 21 years ago. She had no idea what was ahead of her after her life-changing assault. The trauma robbed her of nearly two decades and produced cumulative victimization and trauma. But she is finding her way now—informed by the ACE Study and inspired by the science of hope.

ACEs and Intimate Relationships

There is new research that reinforces the importance of identifying childhood trauma and working through it before you pursue intimate relationships in your life. Golan Shahar and Dana Lassri from Ben Gurion University in Israel have published two studies to look at how childhood trauma and emotional abuse can impact romantic relationships later in life.

College students all completed a questionnaire similar to ACEs. Then, they answered questions about their current romantic relationships. The research team found a clear link between childhood trauma and self-criticism (including negative self-talk). They correlated these with dissatisfaction in a person's romantic relationships. Childhood trauma survivors had lower self-esteem and more symptoms of PTSD. The link between childhood trauma and challenges in intimate relationships is not new, but the self-criticism piece is important new research. People who tend to self-criticize have a more difficult time in intimate relationships. People with childhood trauma and a tendency to criticize themselves and struggle with self-esteem need to increase hope in their lives. Rising hope increases self-esteem and helps counter-act a negative self-image. Professional counseling may also be necessary to help develop new patterns of self-talk and make sure that an intimate partner knows of your challenges and the need for encouragement in these areas.

Limits of the ACE Study

The ACE Study is an excellent tool to capture some of the categories of trauma that children experience in their lives. It also helps explain some of the coping mechanisms that people choose in their adolescent and adult lives. We use the ACE Study to help eliminate the shame and blame that often comes with addiction, mental illness, eating disorders, and unhealthy choices. But the ACE Study has its limits.

The ACE Study does not measure cumulative trauma. Other tools and measuring may be necessary to fully understand the diverse and cumulative types of trauma that someone has suffered. We call this polyvictimization, when someone has experienced different kinds of trauma in childhood and then other types in adulthood. We are currently working with the U.S. Department of Justice on a National Polyvictimization Initiative—studying how to provide the best services in Family Justice Centers where virtually all the survivors (adults and children) coming in the door are polyvictims.

A child sexually abused once will experience trauma from this violation. But a child that is sexually abused hundreds of times will face even more significant impacts and long-term consequences. Repeated abuse can create a state of hypervigilance. Hypervigilance puts the brain in overdrive, releasing chemicals that damage neurodevelopment.

A sexually abused girl, bullied in school, living in community violence who then grows up to be strangled and beaten in an intimate relationship as an adult will have even more complex polyvictimization. The ACE Study does not measure repeated traumatic events in your life before the age of 18 or events after the age of 18.

The ACE Study also does not measure other kinds of adversity that can come from hurricanes, tornados, forest fires, the death of a parent, child, or loved one, a car accident, an illness, a life-threatening situation, being fired from a job, a partner's affair, divorce, war, combat, burglary of your home, and a host of other circumstances.

The ACE Study does not measure vicarious trauma either. Vicarious trauma is experienced by those who may be helping others—such as police officers, firefighters, social workers, doctors, nurses, and many other helping professions. Sometimes the telling of a story of trauma causes vicarious trauma to the hearer of the story.

The original ACE Study did not look at criminality either. It was focused on the health outcomes for primarily white, upper-middle class Kaiser Permanente patients in San Diego. Many other studies are now connecting high ACE Scores with criminality in both adolescence and adulthood. Trauma cultivates the smallest germs of anger in the life of a child. Repeated victimizations turn the germ into a contagious infection of rage that drives mostly men to strangle, rape, and kill. The unmitigated rage of childhood adversity is at the foundation of most murders of women, children, and even police officers across this country. The jails, prisons, and mental health facilities of this country are filled with childhood trauma survivors that never got the help they needed and found a path to rising hope. We will see this in the next chapter.

The Importance of ACE Science in Pursuing Hope

Just like Katie, we all need to understand the ACE Study which is the epidemiology of childhood adversity. It is not just about a number (between 0 and 10) though that is what starts the conversation. It is about how many people experience childhood trauma, how many times they experience it, and what happens to them as a result.

Then, we need to understand how repeated childhood trauma experiences produce toxic stress. This toxic stress damages a child's brain and affects their bodily functions—sometimes for only the short-term but very often for life. We all need to know that toxic stress can literally change the DNA of a human being. This altered

DNA can then be passed on from one generation to the next—traveling from the mother and father to the fetus. Thankfully, though, this is not the end of the story. Hope and resilience can change our brains, improve function, and even heal portions that have been damaged. DNA can be negatively impacted and DNA can be positively impacted! ACEs can negatively impact DNA and hope and resilience and evidence-based activities and practices can positively restore or alter damaged DNA! We will look more at this when we talk later about the engine of hope, the human brain.

Honesty without shame about the way trauma impacts our lives is part of the pathway to hope. Christian's journey reminds us how important reaching out for help is to our futures. Openness about how to mitigate trauma is crucial even if we have experienced its impact for years. Katie is a great role model for many others still lost in shame and pain. Overcoming the bad stuff with the good stuff is our goal. Christian's story at the beginning of the chapter proves that rising hope robs trauma of its power. Christian says that his lasting friendships with other kids and adults with similar experiences helped him release the trauma. He needed to find friends that accepted him even after sharing his emotions before he could really set his goals for the future. ACEs will come up again in this book, but now we understand ACEs and see how they help us contextualize our normal reactions to abnormal things that we experience. This is the beginning of becoming "trauma-informed"—understanding the natural reactions of people to trauma and being able to help them process what has happened to them instead of focusing on what is wrong with them.

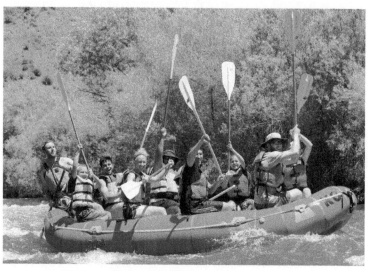

Christian (back right of boat) on the Klamath River
with Camp HOPE America

The ACE Study is a great conversation starter for those dealing with the impacts of childhood trauma. If everyone in this country could learn to talk openly about their ACE Scores without shame or blame, we would have far more authentic conversations about our lives, struggles, and how rising hope can change our lives. The sooner we can make it OK for adults and children to talk about their ACEs, the sooner we can begin the conversation about hope and resiliency and ways to take back our power from trauma.

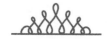

Chapter 10

Sometimes It is Too Late for Hope

"Abandon all hope, you who enter here."
—Dante's Sign at the Gates of Hell

Devon

Devon Patrick Kelley was discharged from the Air Force in 2014 for "bad conduct" after being prosecuted for domestic violence and child abuse. He fractured a child's skull and strangled his wife. The Air Force gave him a break, letting him avoid a more serious charge that could have put him in prison for much longer and would have given him a dishonorable discharge. He only spent a year in jail for a rage-filled assault on his step-son and wife. And it was not the first time he had assaulted or threatened a woman, child, or animal. In fact, he even threatened to kill his military superiors and ended up escaping from a mental health facility. Under the federal felony statute in the Violence Against Women Act, he could have gotten ten years in prison for a first offense. But not in the Air Force. A year in jail—typical for a misdemeanor offense in many states—was his only sentence. This caused him only to lose one rank and face a bad conduct discharge. After his conviction, the Air Force violated federal law by not notifying the FBI of his conviction— giving him another break.

Because his military conviction was never reported to the FBI, Devon Patrick Kelley was able to buy assault rifles and handguns between 2016 and 2017 without any red flags in his background check. On November 5, 2017, he showed up outside the First Baptist Church of Sutherland Springs, Texas, looking to kill his mother-in-law, and opened fire. Then, he went into the church and committed the largest mass murder in a church in modern American history. He killed 26 and injured 20 including children, entire families, and elderly men and women. After he changed Sutherland Springs forever, he fled the church and eventually killed himself while being chased by a good Samaritan intervenor, Johnny Langendorf, who helped bring Kelley's murderous rage to an end.

The full story of Devon Patrick Kelley's childhood trauma and the impact of trauma during his military enlistment has never been told. But seeing his rage and understanding how the failure to aggressively intervene by many facilitated a mass murderer's action is important. Sometimes when we don't intervene in time, time runs out.

Devon Patrick Kelley is not the only mass murderer where it became too late for hope. Every day the news is filled with stories of those where rage, despair, resentment, and low hope produce life-ending tragedy. His story illustrates the relationship between mass shootings in this country, high ACE scores, and domestic violence. Domestic violence and childhood trauma form the "why" of America's mass murder problem.

There is also another marker in Kelley's journey that also should have told us his rage had grown into murderous intent. Devon Patrick Kelley was a strangler. In the Air Force court martial documents, when he was prosecuted for child abuse and domestic violence in 2012, they only referred to it as "choking." He "choked" his wife. Choking is when food gets caught in your throat. When Kelley placed his hands around his wife's neck, he was committing the felony crime of strangulation.

Strangulation is external pressure to the neck that blocks air or blood flow even for seconds. When Kelley put his hands around a woman's neck, he was telling people he was a killer and no one paid attention. Once a woman is strangled, she is 750% more likely to later be killed by that man. No one treated his strangulation as seriously as it deserved to be treated. He needed the science of hope and treatment for his trauma issues long before he was standing outside the First Baptist Church in Sutherland Springs.

The work of Alliance for HOPE International and its allied organizations focus on helping trauma exposed children. But they also focus heavily, through their Training Institute on Strangulation Prevention, on men who strangle women.

Men who strangle women are the most dangerous men on the planet. The mass murderers are domestic violence offenders. But more specifically, they are stranglers. The founder of the Training Institute on Strangulation Prevention, Gael Strack, calls strangulation "the last warning shot" before a murder or mass murder. Gael and Casey are focused on documenting, investigating, and prosecuting non-fatal strangulation cases successfully before the murder or mass murder occurs.

Domestic violence stranglers, usually after being trauma-exposed children, are the why of mass murders and guns are the how. Rage-filled, violent men should not be allowed access to assault rifles, handguns, or any other firearms of any kind. Our research shows the "how" to stop stranglers — holding offenders accountable for domestic violence strangulation and sexual assault strangulation before they later commit a mass murder. Then, we need to take away their guns.

This is why we also advocate for bringing agencies together in communities to create Family Justice/Multi-Agency Centers, that we have also touched on earlier, where survivors can get comprehensive services in one place. We will look more closely about the success of these Centers later in the book—they are beacons of hope. Offenders face greater accountability from multi-disciplinary teams of police, prosecutors, advocates, probation/parole officers, and other professionals. It is the 'Power of We' in doing both prevention and intervention work with adult and child survivors in a trauma-informed, holistic approach. Our research proves the "how" — that Family Justice Centers increase hope in the lives of adult and child survivors and produce better accountability for offenders.

In America, we raise our criminals at home and we must focus on breaking the cycle of generational violence with the children exposed to trauma. But much earlier than that, they need help as children. This is why the Alliance runs the largest camping and mentoring program in the country for children exposed to domestic violence that we have touched on in this book. Camp HOPE America is one of the how's — the largest camping and mentoring program ever created to help children impacted by domestic violence. We can love them and change their destinies at 10 or wait and debate motives and causes after mass murders when they are adults. It is our choice. Our published research, shared in the next few chapters, proves you can change the destinies of rage-filled boys before they become rage-filled men and help girls avoid a lifetime of victimization by increasing hope and giving them pathways to a life without abuse. Even if you don't work in or connect often to the criminal justice system, our write up of our criminal justice research is good for you to know. You should be demanding trauma-informed, hope-centered work in your local criminal justice system if you want to deter the terrible tragedy of Sutherland Springs from ever happening in your community.

The more you understand the science of hope, the more critically you will read news stories and coverage of mass shooters and terrorists. You will start evaluating how well trauma and ACEs are covered by reporters and news outlets. With our understanding of ACEs and trauma, the story of Las Vegas shooter Stephen Paddock presents an opportunity to evaluate how both the media and the FBI covered and investigated a trauma-impacted child who became a mass murderer.

As you read the story below, ask yourself whether Paddock seems like a person with high hope or low hope. Do you think he had rage, despair, apathy about even living? Do you think finding motive is the right approach or should the FBI be thinking more about his mental state over the course of life? And note how his brother tried to feign shock at what happened.

Stephen

Professional gambler Stephen Paddock, the Las Vegas shooter, who killed 59 and injured 527 people at a country western concert in the largest mass shooting in modern history had a profound childhood trauma history but the FBI and even his brother have ignored it. Right after the carnage, his brother Eric said "an asteroid fell from the sky" because Stephen gave no indications "at all" that he was on this pathway according to his brother. The FBI and an army of Nevada law enforcement professionals immediately began searching for a "motive"—that has remained elusive. Everyone wants to find reason and logic in this heinous, unimaginable crime. They want to explain why Paddock attacked 22,000 innocent country western music concert goers with automatic weapons from the 32nd Floor of the Mandalay Bay Hotel. So far, we only get to blame "bump stocks" and argue about the 2nd Amendment. Time will tell what else they discover but we already know enough to make some sense of the rage-filled actions of Paddock. The answer is connected to the ACE Study. Once we all understand ACEs, we won't buy the lie that "an asteroid fell from the sky."

Paddock's childhood trauma doesn't give us a traditional motive. But it does give us an explanation for the genesis of a mass murderer. The higher an ACE score the greater the likelihood of adult criminality and rage-motivated behavior. As we have seen, an ACE Score of 4 or greater is correlated with everything from mental illness, to sociopathic and psychopathic behavior, to drug and alcohol abuse.

Fact: Most of the mass murderers/shooters, homegrown terrorists, prison inmates, rapists, and violent criminals in this country grew up in homes with some mix of child abuse, domestic violence, neglect, verbal and emotional abuse, and drug and/or alcohol abuse. The ACEs of childhood produce the rage and criminality of adulthood.

Based on what we know so far, with very limited information on Paddock's childhood, we know he was verbally, emotionally, and violently abused by his brother Bruce, abandoned by his psychopathic, mentally ill father at age 7, the product of divorced parents, regularly subjected to fear of violence and abuse in his home growing up, and the son of an incarcerated father. This gives Paddock an ACE Score of at least 7 and dramatically increases the likelihood that he would grow up with unmitigated rage and chronic mental health issues. We don't know the whole story yet but he was at least verbally and emotionally, if not physically abusive, to the intimate partners in his life and struggled with depression. Our guess is we will find all kinds of other anti-social behavior when the whole story is told. He lacked attachment to virtually anyone—no close friends have come forward from anywhere—and he was obsessed with possessing and firing military style weapons without out any interest in hunting, target shooting, skeet shooting, or recreational gun use with friends or social acquaintances.

It is easy to say "Who cares? He was a killer and he made choices that other people don't make even when bad things have happened to them." True. When acts like the Las Vegas mass shooting happen—no one has any sympathy for the killer and no one wants to hear someone was abused as a child. Fair enough. Many grow up with violence and abuse and abandonment in their lives and they don't become infamous mass murderers. But virtually all the mass murderers have high ACE Scores. Virtually all radicalized American terrorists have high ACE scores. What is the difference then? Those that don't suffer the documented impacts of a high ACE score have many mitigating factors in their lives—caring friends, mentors that help them set goals and then achieve those goals, strong social support, healthy relationships with other adults, and mental health support as needed. They also likely find their way to higher hope. This truth means we must invest in trauma-exposed children to prevent the next generation of mass murderers. We must learn to produce rising hope in the youngest trauma victims as soon as we can possibly access them after trauma in their lives. Stephen Paddock had none of these mitigating forces in his life as a child or as an adult. There is little doubt he was a rage-filled, low hope man. It is not an excuse. It is not a complete explanation. It does not provide the "motive" we all want in the Las Vegas mass shooting. But don't buy the lie that an "asteroid fell from the sky."

In America, we raise our criminals at home. Most likely, Devon Patrick Kelley's rage and Stephen Paddock's psychopathic mental processes began in their homes growing up or soon thereafter. There is little doubt in our minds that Kelley had a significant ACE score and Paddock's was clearly high. The media has never talked about their childhood trauma histories. Not all mass shooters grow up in abusive homes and not all abused children become mass shooters. But low hope (rage + despair) in both these men turned them into uncontrollable killing machines and childhood adversity was likely the birth place of their rage and despair. Then, violence against women in adulthood spurred it forward. It also produces virtually every mass shooter in the country.

For many years, Sea World in San Diego hosted the Shamu Show. Children often loved sitting in the front rows because when Shamu jumped the splash would hit everyone in the lower rows. Signs warned viewers of the show to stay back from the pool tank unless they wanted to get soaked by Shamu's actions. Many children of trauma grow up to repeat the generational cycle of violence and, in some cases, the "splash zone" of their rage produces mass murder. Most mass shooters are childhood trauma survivors and domestic violence offenders where there has been no mitigation or intervention. The evidence is clear that nine out of ten of the deadliest mass shootings in modern America were perpetrated by men with histories of violence against women, threatened violence against women, or disparaging conduct toward women. All nine of the killers also had a history of childhood adversity that clearly laid the foundation for what was to come in their lives. Devon Patrick Kelley and Stephen Paddock are both on the list.

High ACE Scores and Cop Killers

Justin

Police officer Justin Terney was 22 years old. He had been on the Tecumseh Police Department just over a year. His dream in life was to be a K-9 officer. He was about to start training and the department had just ordered the puppy to begin the long process of training and bonding for Justin and the dog.

On March 26, 2017, Justin pulled over a car with a female driver because a tail light was out. It was a routine traffic stop. He approached the car and asked for license and registration. The woman gave him her information. There was also a male passenger in the car. He asked for the man's identification as well. The man said he did not have any and gave him a name. Justin checked the names and quickly determined that the man had given a fake name. He called for back-up. Justin asked the man to get out of the car and confronted him about his actual name. The man instead bolted and ran from the car. Justin gave chase as the man ran into the bushes and jumped a fence. Justin jumped the fence as well and used his Taser to try to stop the man.

The Taser did not work. Right after Justin fired the Taser, the man pulled a gun and shot Officer Justin Terney four times. Justin returned fire and hit the man three times. Other officers subdued the suspect and paramedics soon arrived to transport both men to the hospital. Justin lived through the night but died of his injuries on the morning of March 27, 2017. His killer survived.

Justin's killer was Byron Shepard. Bryon Shepard had a history of domestic violence including strangulation assault against women. He had faced little accountability in the criminal justice system for his crimes. His journey through childhood trauma produced a rage-filled man who taxpayers will now fund to spend the rest of his life in prison. Justin will never become a K-9 officer or live the life he had dreamed of and was pursuing with high hope and determination. Justin's puppy was delivered to begin K-9 training at the Tecumseh Police Department just days after his funeral.

As we have seen, the majority of all mass shootings are committed by childhood trauma survivors and occur in the context of domestic violence situations. The other deeply disturbing finding this past year by Alliance for HOPE International is the fact that the majority of all police officers killed in the United States are killed by men with a history of domestic violence. Officer Justin Terney is only one of dozens of officers killed each year by men with a history of unmitigated childhood trauma and an adult history of violence against women usually including strangulation of a woman.

The FBI annually releases statistics about law enforcement officers killed in the line of duty. The 2016 Statistics for Law Enforcement Officers killed in the line of duty by intentional felonious acts were similar to previous years. We honor, remember, and mourn each and every officer and remember their children, spouses, and family members who have experienced such heartbreak and loss.

We assisted the staff of Alliance for HOPE International in conducting an initial scan of the Internet-available criminal history of each law enforcement officer killer identified in 2017. The 2017 data is very revealing. Nearly 80% of all killers of law enforcement officers in this country have a domestic violence history locatable on the Internet and 20% have a strangulation assault history. This is data we have identified without any access to full criminal histories and without interviews of each killer's prior intimate partners. We have little doubt that the actual percentages are dramatically higher than we have found on the Internet.

We see three major issues that must be addressed. First, the annual FBI data analysis minimizes domestic violence by calling it a "domestic disturbance". It should be called "domestic violence" which more accurately describes the crimes occurring when officers arrive at the scene (and later die). Second, the FBI data and analysis misleads the public and law enforcement officers by ignoring the significance of relationship history of the killers. The rage of a man who beats and strangles a woman is the same rage of a man that kills a police officer.

Third, the FBI must produce better analysis if we are going to focus on the real killers of women and police officers in this country. The real killers are men who strangle (choke) women. If a man strangles a woman, he is 750% more likely to later kill her. We need to focus far more energy on homicide prevention by going after the stranglers in this country.

Stranglers are the cop killers of America. We are failing law enforcement officers across this country by not educating them on the correlation between domestic violence perpetration and intentional homicide of law enforcement officers.

Devon Patrick Kelley, Stephen Paddock and Bryon Shepard needed rising hope long before they became killers. They needed intervention as children and teens that was never offered. They needed pathways to address their trauma issues early in their lives. And the day came for Kelley and so many others in Sutherland Springs, Texas, for Paddock and hundreds of country western fans in Vegas, and for Officer Justin Terney in Oklahoma, when it was too late for hope to rise. The killers abandoned all hope at the gates of hell.

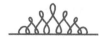

Chapter 11

Great Leaders, Visionaries, and Gifted People with Demons

"Most great men or women have their demons. They have pain, heartbreak, and even rage that sometimes drives them. Usually, they have high hope too in some or all areas of their lives that preserves them and sustains them through the darkness. But hope is no panacea. We need to be honest that sometimes hope even runs out in those that have been sustained by it for most of their lives."
—Casey Gwinn

Bill

Bill grew up in Seattle, Washington. He was the youngest of eight children. His father, Gardner, was an apartment builder and contractor. He was bigger than life—a community leader, church deacon, and driven man. His mom Mabel was a homemaker. She was a firm but strong woman. Bill learned about relationships, love, parenting, and commitment from his parents.

Mabel married Gardner soon after his first wife died during childbirth. She had never been married, but she was taken with this young widower with his three small children. Gardner was a businessman with dreams and aspirations and a broken heart after the death of his first wife.

Gardner courted Mabel; they fell in love and soon married. Mabel wanted to care for Gardner and his sons, but she also wanted her own children. Within two years, she was pregnant. Over the course of the next 12 years, she gave birth to five children of her own. Bill was the last of those five children that Gardner and Mabel would have together.

Gardner was not abusive with Mabel at first. He was a firm disciplinarian with the children, but he did not raise a hand toward her until later in their marriage. His anger and rage were potent. No child ever wanted to cross him. The consequences were swift and unequivocal.

Bill would later recall his father's tongue lashings, name calling, and physical abuse. His older sister would much later recall ushering Bill out of the room when their mom and dad began to argue. Bill remembered his dad throwing things at his mother. He remembered his sister walking him to a bedroom and turning the radio up so they could not hear the arguments in the other room. And Bill remembered, like it was yesterday, his father saying over and over, "Quit your crying or I'll give you something to cry about."

The verbal and emotional abuse in Gardner's home was consistent but not constant. There were good times too—making it harder to sort out the wrong from the right. The children grew up not knowing that healthy families did not function like the family ruled by Gardner. They grew up thinking their family was like all others.

All of Gardner's abusive ways were never fully documented. Mabel took most of her secrets to the grave and never talked about Gardner's rage and violence in the home. He was publicly a man of honor and prestige. Buildings bore his name and business and political leaders feared and revered him.

But the worst abuse that Bill suffered was not the verbal and emotional abuse or even the whippings that came with a vengeance. The worst abuse was a quiet, daily punch to the head that Bill suffered from his father. Why his father targeted him for the closed fist wakeup call every day, Bill would never know. "Wee Willy Wee, wake up." And his father would rap him on the side of the head with a closed fist.

Bill survived Gardner's home with a loving mother and cheerleaders in many areas of his life. He learned to play tennis and ski. He went off to college and excelled in academics and sports. He fell in love, found his passion in the world of Christian ministry, went to seminary, and became a youth minister. He had learned the value of hard work from his father and he had a special sense of calling to help kids as he worked as a youth pastor in Pasadena at Lake Avenue Congregational Church.

One day, he had a dream that two men in suits would show up and ask him to be the director of a growing Christian camp called Mount Hermon in the Santa Cruz

Mountains of Northern California. He told his wife about the dream and they both wondered if it was real.

Two weeks later, two men in suits walked into his office and asked him to come be the Director of Mount Hermon Conference Center. He was only 28 years old. He and his wife packed up their apartment and their two young children and moved to Northern California.

Bill thrived in his new role. He was an extrovert, a dreamer, a visionary, and a driven man like his father. The camp thrived and grew under his leadership. Bill rose to be the President of Christian Camping International and had an illustrious career in serving others, promoting the power of camping, and making a difference in the world.

Bill and his wife, Colette, had two more children and settled in to raise their family in the 1960's and 1970s. Bill never hit his wife like his father had hit his mother. But his rage often resulted in "discipline" of his children and verbal and emotional abuse that would play itself out for decades in their adult lives. He was not a monster though. There were many good times in the family as the children grew up along with the bad times. He was, at times, affirming and encouraging. He was present and engaged. He attended his children's sporting events and celebrated their accomplishments.

But there were demons. Not until the 1980s did it become apparent that Bill was bipolar. He struggled deeply with suicidal ideation for a number of years after his mental health issues worsened. Subsequent research on head trauma, would eventually point to traumatic brain injury from being punched in the head as the likely cause of his chemical imbalance and bipolar disorder. Bill's mental health issues eventually landed him in psychiatric lock-up units and subjected his family to profoundly unpredictable patterns of behavior. A great man and visionary would struggle with his demons from childhood for most of his life.

Bill was a great leader and visionary who never fully overcame his battle with childhood trauma. The journey through mental illness for Bill Gwinn shaped Casey's life. His dad's abuse as a child was repeated in some but not all ways in Casey's life and the lives of his brother and sisters. But there was also high hope in Bill Gwinn. He was goal-oriented and strategic in his thinking as he built Mount Hermon, spent decades as a pastor, and advised camps and Christian ministries across the United States. He navigated through profound obstacles in achieving great things in his life. Most people are not all good or all bad. Most are not high hope all the time or low hope all the time.

Casey's dad never took his ACE score. He never even publicly admitted that he suffered from bipolar disorder, depression, mental illness, or the impacts of childhood trauma. But we can say with certainty that he had a high ACE score.

Bill Gwinn would have also scored high on hope for most of his adult life. High hope likely carried him through many struggles. Even with times of depression, suicidal ideation, and difficulty, he had a remarkable life of helping others and serving his God.

Rick Snyder and Bill Gwinn would have been friends. Those driven by high hope are drawn to others like them. Visionaries and leaders often connect with other visionaries and leaders.

Bill Gwinn had a minor heart attack on April 14, 2009. He was taken to Palm Desert Regional Medical Center. The doctors said a stent could be placed that would give him many more years of life, but his kidneys were unstable—likely from 30 years of lithium to treat his bipolar disorder. They worked to stabilize his kidneys for two days. The stent to address blockage in his heart was not put in place in the interim.

Casey visited his dad on the evening of April 16th. His dad had high hope and was excited to be able to think about new goals and was planning to feel better after heart surgery in a few days. But his dad also seemed to have some sense of the brevity of life. He asked Casey to promise he would take care of his mom, handle all the family finances, and take a book about the history of Mount Hermon from his dad's home office to the current Director of the Conference Center. "I will take care of the bills. I will take Roger the book. I promise I will help mom with everything she needs, Dad." Then, his dad became more serious. "I am sorry for the times I have failed you, son. I am sorry for a lot of things I have done in my life. I hope you will forgive me." Bill Gwinn began to cry. Casey did not hesitate. "I forgive you, Dad. It's all in the past. You did the best you could. I love you." Casey kissed his dad on the forehead and left the hospital to get some rest.

Bill Gwinn would never have heart surgery. Casey would never see him alive again. Not in this life.

The next morning, April 17, 2009, Bill had a massive heart attack while in ICU at Palm Desert Regional Medical Center. They tried to resuscitate him for 20 minutes including using a defibrillator on him three times as his wife Colette sobbed in the corner of the room. But Bill was gone. Later, a nurse told Casey his dad fixated on a point on the ceiling and never stopped staring at it until they pronounced him dead. Casey said, "My dad was not fixated on the ceiling. He was looking into eternity. It was time for the pain to end and he knew where he was going." The nurse stared back,

"Oh, you must be religious." Casey was kind and soft with her. "No, just hopeful. So very hopeful that I will see my dad again one day."

Not the Only One

Bill Gwinn was not the only one. There are many other great leaders, visionaries, actors, actresses, athletes, business icons, and other high achievers in modern times and throughout history that have been high hope human beings much of the time while still tormented by the impacts of a high ACE score. There is so little general public discussion about ACEs that few of their stories have ever been fully told. In the years to come, it is our prayer that many more will tell their stories of childhood trauma. A high ACE score is not an excuse for bad conduct, but is an explanation. We would like to see many more explanations. Many more explanations would help those survivors find more help and support for their secret pain.

The landscape of history is littered with the lives of many who have struggled deeply with depression and pain related to childhood trauma and abuse. Some end up committing suicide. The most rage-filled end up committing murder-suicide. We talked to multiple women whose spouses took their own lives and they each said something very similar to this: "He tried to keep his pain behind a door in his mind, but finally he couldn't stop it from coming out from behind the door." Many live with pain behind a door they wish would never open. And the list is not restricted to great leaders, visionaries, or the gifted and talented. According to the World Health Organization, 800,000 people take their own lives every year and millions attempt to take their own lives. This book is not focused on the multiple causes of suicide, but the majority of all suicides trace their causal roots back to childhood trauma and very low hope. Many of their childhood stories, however, have never been told.

The relationship between suicidal ideation, suicide attempts/completions, and childhood trauma is undeniable. The risk of suicide attempts for those with high ACE scores is 51 times higher in children and adolescents and 30 times higher in adults compared to those with a zero ACE score. This order of magnitude is just as high as the relationship between using opioids and childhood trauma! 64% of all suicide attempts by adults and 80% of suicide attempts by adolescents have been connected to ACEs. Growing up with child abuse and domestic violence is bad, but the greatest predictor of suicide is not physical abuse, it is emotional abuse.

The American military has been dealing with an estimated 22 suicide deaths per day in recent years. The military does not talk about it but two published studies have found that childhood trauma is dramatically higher in those military members who commit suicide than those who do not. The prevalence of suicide in the military is stunning but not much higher than the national average. The CDC estimates that an American takes his or her own life every 16 minutes. Many at risk for suicide really do want to live and their suicidal signals are their way of asking for help. The majority of suicide attempts are the culmination of varied triggers. Triggers may connect to a broken relationship, financial problems, or legal issues. The primary trigger may be loss of a child, parent, or spouse. Sometimes the primary trigger appears to be low self-esteem, rejection, drug or alcohol abuse, or the suicide of a family member or friend. But when you peel away the layers, there is often childhood trauma and low hope.

One woman we interviewed, Mary, said that her husband's suicide was his effort to escape the pain of his childhood trauma. *"He (John) was not trying to kill himself. His death was like people jumping out of windows at 9/11. They were not trying to die. They were trying to get away from the flames. John was not trying to kill himself. He was trying to get away from the pain."* John had never publicly disclosed his childhood trauma experiences. His triggers that led to his suicide connected to depression. But don't be misled, at the core was the pain of childhood trauma.

In recent years, the list of high profile people from all professions that have struggled with depression and then have taken their own lives is long. It includes Robin Williams (actor), Gia Allemand (actress), Mike Awesome (professional wrestler), Nikki Bacharach (daughter of Burt Bacharach), Simone Battle (singer), Jeremy Black (artist), Eduardo Bonvallet (Chilean World Cup Soccer Player), Jovan Belcher (NFL Player, Kansas City Chiefs), Dave Duerson (NFL Player, Chicago Bears), Vince Foster (Deputy White House Counsel), Aaron Hernandez (NFL Player, New England Patriots), Nicolas Hughes (Biologist), Mike Kelley (American artist), Harry Lew (U.S. Marine), Andrew Martinez (U.C. Berkeley's "Naked Guy"), Jason Moss (attorney), Jeret "Speedy" Peterson (Olympic medalist skier), Roy Raymond (Founder of Victoria's Secret), Roh Moo-hyun (President of South Korea), Junior Seau (NFL Player, San Diego Chargers), Jean Stein (author), Sawyer Sweeten (Actor, Everybody Loves Raymond), Amanda Todd (bullied Canadian high school student), Edwin Valero (boxer), Bob Welch (Fleetwood Mac singer), Jack Wishna (President and CEO, CP Capital), and Bill Zeller (Developer of myTunes). And many others. Most of them experienced childhood and subsequent adult trauma in one form or another yet most of their full childhood stories have never been told. Many of them did amazing things in their lives—setting goals and finding pathways to their goals for many years before hope ran out.

Hope Heroes Everywhere

There are celebrities and high profile public figures that have honestly shared their childhood trauma and have modeled how to overcome it. Casey was inspired many years ago by Oprah Winfrey when she profiled Casey's work at the San Diego Family Justice Center on her show in January 2003. Oprah Winfrey has been a powerful role model to so many women, girls, men, and boys that have experienced trauma and abuse. She has told the truth of her trauma. There are many others as well that come to mind—Tyler Perry endured beatings with an extension cord and growing up with an alcoholic father. Nicki Minaj grew up with a drug addicted father and lived in a constant state of hypervigilance as a child, fearing her dad would kill her and her mother. Rapper DMX has shared harrowing stories of being beaten with braided extension cords and once losing teeth from a beating with a broom handle. Mary Blige has courageously talked about being sexually molested at five years old.

Eleanor Roosevelt many years ago and, more recently, Bill Clinton, have talked about their journeys through childhood trauma. Rapper Eminem has talked about growing up without a father and facing bullying and other impacts of growing up poor in public housing. The list goes on and on of those hope heroes that have overcome their trauma and have gone on to great successes in their lives including actors Dylan McDermott, Chevy Chase, Woody Harelson, and Queen Latifah. The well-known names of those who have been willing to be transparent and have overcome by pursuing their dreams relentlessly goes on and on—Tina Turner, Gloria Steinem, Antwone Fisher, evangelist Joyce Meyer, Carlos Santana, Fantasia, and Duane Lee Chapman (Dog the Bounty Hunter). We love the high hope of Eve Ensler who has taken her pain and used it to raise awareness in so many ways including the wildly successful *Vagina Monologues*. Ashley Judd recently disclosed she has an ACE score of 9. She has connected her success to the power of hope: "When I needed it, one person extended the hand of hope and help to me. It saved me." Ashley and so many others join our list of hope heroes as they share what happened to them openly and honestly.

Inocente

When Inocente was 11 years old, and living out of a car in San Diego with her mom and brother, her mom announced after a cold, shivering night without a home, "I want us to go jump from the Coronado Bridge. I can't take it anymore. I want the pain to end." Inocente refused. She had dreams and goals. She had started painting in an art program and discovered her incredible gift. She talked her mom out of it. Two years later, even while still homeless, the documentary of Inocente's journey won an Academy Award. In

2016, Yesenia Aceves, from the Camp HOPE America team, reached out to Inocente to ask if she would do an art project with our children. Inocente agreed without hesitation. Days later, Inocente showed up at Yesenia's office and carried with her two small 4 X 6 photographs of Inocente attending Camp HOPE San Diego when she was 9 and 10 years old. Though Camp HOPE wasn't measuring hope back in those days, her camping experience was the beginning of her hopes and dreams in her own life. Rising hope saved Inocente's life even if we didn't know that is what we were doing.

The art program that helped Inocente doesn't measure hope. But the reality is that Inocente's rising hope in her life at age 11 helped keep her mom from taking her own life and ending Inocente's. The power of hope in a child was the difference between life and death in her despair-filled mom.

We Honor Those Who Battle Demons

We honor Bill Gwinn here along with many other great visionaries and dreamers in mind who have battled their demons, overcome profound childhood trauma, and accomplished great things in their lives. We don't honor them because they are all perfect. We don't honor them because they have never hurt those they loved the most. We honor them because they are great men and women with feet of clay who have refused to let the trauma of their ACEs define them.

Like many great women and men with pain and millions of Americans, Bill Gwinn struggled with depression. Most of those listed above have as well. Remember the high likelihood of depression in high ACE score adults that we saw earlier? If you have an ACE score of 4, the likelihood of suffering from depression goes up 300% as an adult. The higher your ACE score, the higher that percentage goes.

Depression can be dealt with as so many do after coming to grips with the battle. Depression is not the opposite of hope. Depression is sometimes a medical issue that can be treated, but must never be demeaned or minimized. It is also commonly the result of untreated and often undisclosed childhood and adult trauma. We will see more obstacles to hope later in this book, but it is important to acknowledge that when we meet someone struggling with demons, it does not mean they cannot find their way to high hope—in fact, high hope may be the thing that has sustained them for most of their lives.

Bill Gwinn's journey shaped his son, who would one day devote his life to making the world safer for children. When a childhood trauma survivor ultimately takes his own life, his death does not demean the power of hope. It proves it. With all he battled in his life, he should have died young. We honor those here who have been unable to keep the pain "behind the door." When a great visionary, leader, thinker, or powerful leader's life ends in suicide, their deaths challenge us to tell the truth about our lives and our families. We have found that studying the lives of those who have taken their own lives has mentored us in life and in death. Childhood trauma is not an *excuse* for the unhealthy decisions that Bill Gwinn and many others, including us, have made. But it is an *explanation* and helps us think deeply about the need for honesty and transparency and the courage to share what many of us keep "behind the door."

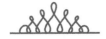

Chapter 12

Lessons Learned from Abused Kids

"Camp HOPE is a place where you really learn what hope is. It is a place to get rid of all those hard feelings you have inside you."
—**Zach**, Age 10

Gemma

Gemma's first memory is being whipped with a switch by her mother in Mexico. She was three years old. Her mother had been gone for months in Acapulco and left her with a caretaker. The day she came back, Gemma was beaten because her mom found her without shoes on her feet. She would live with her mom's violence for years—beatings with a stick, a belt, a wire, a coat hanger, in the name of discipline. Years later, Gemma would look back and say, "My mom's 'discipline' of me was fueled by her own rage from being beaten when she was a child." But another abuser would come into Gemma's life.

When Gemma was five she was brought illegally to the United States by her mother and her mom's boyfriend. He was an alcoholic and an abuser. Her mom told her the man was her father. For years, Gemma did not know any different. At age 5, Gemma began to sense his presence in her bedroom at night. It would last for nearly a decade of her childhood. He molested her hundreds of times until she was 13 years old. Gemma's stepdad was deported when she was 13, not for molesting her but for dealing drugs.

She still calls his deportation one of the "best days of my life." The violence and abuse at times left Gemma depressed and dark, but there were mitigating forces in her life and many opportunities to set goals and pursue pathways forward. By age 14, Gemma was starting high school but confesses today she was "mostly driven by anger toward my stepdad." She is smart, articulate, and organized. She first attended Camp HOPE at age 13 and found friends, inspiration, and goals for her life. She said she wanted to be a biologist at her first campfire when we asked what kids wanted to do when they grew up.

Gemma's mom wanted her to have the educational opportunities she did not have herself growing up. She found a willing friend and got Gemma a mailing address that would get her into better primary and secondary schools, including a high school with a strong science program. Gemma found other smart, driven high schoolers and soon enrolled into the school's four-year Biomedical Science program. She excelled in science and math and did well in high school. Each summer she and her brother attended Camp HOPE America and found encouragement, friends, and possibilities for the future. At 16, she described her motivation in life. "I am driven by my anger. I know it looks like I am just driven in a good way but if you put me in a room with my stepdad today and put a knife between us—I would grab the knife and stab him as many times as I could until you stopped me." Camp HOPE helped her find ways to turn her anger into power and let go of some of the anger and unforgiveness that could have destroyed her like a cancer.

Gemma is a so-called "Dreamer"—brought to the United States without legal status by a parent without legal status. It only compounded the trauma as she grew up—realizing the risk she faced of being deported from the only country she has ever really called home. Working with Camp HOPE America, Gemma got her legal residency status this past year.

Gemma enrolled in college last year and now says she wants to be a lawyer instead of a biologist. The truth: She can be anyone and anything she wants to be in life. She still has bouts of depression, suicidal ideation, and anger but she is learning to talk about it, work through issues with a counselor, advocate for herself, and share her story with others. She will also tell anyone that asks that the pathway is not linear. There are ups and downs. There are good days and bad days. Her negative self-talk sometimes wins the day. But at other times, she can see the truth: She is smart, gifted, beautiful, powerful, and destined to do great things with her life. She is an introvert that struggles with relationships, but she is also incredibly gifted in working with girls that have experienced violence and abuse. Gemma is still experiencing in many ways the impact of generational trauma as well. Gemma's mom would likely score a 10 on the ACE Scale. Gemma's mom needed

Camp HOPE many years ago in her own life. But Gemma is learning that her pain, her challenges, even her anger are natural and normal reactions to what she has overcome.

Gemma has been high on willpower and waypower for most of her life. She does still tend, at times, toward depression and discouragement like many children and teens impacted by child abuse and domestic violence. But she is learning the science of hope and now more consciously focuses on ways to maintain or increase both her willpower and her waypower. She is a high hope young woman with a bright future even amidst the normal reactions to her profound trauma over the early years of her life.

The Risk of Child Maltreatment and Hope

Our research, and that of other researchers, demonstrates that targeted interventions and personal strategies can increase the hopeful capacity of those who have experienced trauma, including parents now at-risk for abusing their children just like they were abused. For example, Chan surveyed almost 200 parents who were identified at moderate to high risk for committing child abuse and neglect. These parents were identified by the child protection system and receiving treatment services to reduce their risk of offending. In the child maltreatment literature, one of the significant predictors for abuse of children by parents is parenting stress. His study found that hope mediated the relationship between parenting stress and the parent-child relationship. Put plainly, the negative effects of parenting stress were mitigated when parents' Hope scores increased. Treatment professionals rated the progress of the parent's independent of the parent Hope scores. Then, he compared the progress of the parents with rising Hope scores. What he found was that 90% of these parents who were identified as making significant progress toward positive parenting also scored higher on hope.

In another study, we conducted longitudinal (over time) research on a home visit program for parents at high risk for child abuse and neglect. Within six months of treatment, we found that improving a parent's hope significantly improved the parent-child relationship quality in the areas of empathy, discipline, and child empowerment. Rising hope produced powerful, positive outcomes for the parents and for the children.

Chan's research team also conducted a nationwide study on child abuse pediatricians. They were interested in the relationship between compassion fatigue and burnout in this high stress field. Professionals who work around childhood trauma and domestic violence are often vulnerable to psychological difficulties such as debilitating anxiety and stress associated with reliving the trauma they have seen and heard from those they are trying to help. These effects are often referred to as compassion fatigue, vicarious trauma, and/or secondary traumatic stress and can lead to high levels of emotional exhaustion and disengagement (burnout). While the study found higher levels of compassion fatigue were related to burnout among these child abuse pediatricians, it also found that increasing hope mitigated the negative effects of compassion fatigue.

Camp HOPE America

Approximately 18+ million children are exposed to domestic violence in the United States each year. These children are likely to experience higher levels of depression, anxiety, fear, and social isolation than children that are not witnessing domestic violence in their homes. A growing body of research is also showing that children who are exposed to domestic violence are also more likely to experience physical abuse themselves. The result of these traumatic experiences for children is an increased level of aggression and violence. These children are more likely to enter the juvenile justice system and have an increased propensity to perpetuate the cycle of domestic violence as survivors or perpetrators. In response to this crisis, Casey has developed Camp HOPE America, the first camping and mentoring program in the United States focused on children impacted by domestic violence and related child abuse.

Camp HOPE America is a program of Alliance for HOPE International which operates under Casey's leadership. The activities and curriculum for Camp HOPE America are built around the science of hope. The goal of Camp HOPE America is to raise Hope scores in the lives of traumatized children to mitigate the damage from their exposure to domestic violence. The research is very clear that children impacted by domestic violence are more likely to repeat it as teens and adults. They are less likely to graduate from high school or college. And they are far more likely to experience lifelong impacts including rage, drug and alcohol addiction, depression, sexual assault as adults, and mental illness.

We have found that by teaching children about goal setting, motivation, and pathways thinking that we can help them more consciously set goals and then achieve them. When we do this, their Hope scores rise and improved outcomes in their lives follow.

In 2017, we published a peer-reviewed journal article investigating increases in children's hope and character strength because of Camp HOPE's intentional hope-centered approach with children exposed to domestic violence. With a smaller subsample, we investigated the prevalence of ACE scores among the children. As seen in the Table below, the national prevalence of ACE indicates that about 64% of the population has an ACE score of one or higher and that about 12-13% have four or more adverse childhood experiences. For the Camp HOPE children, we found that 100% have an ACE score of one or higher with 80% having a score of four or higher. We found these children have significantly higher trauma scores (Average 5.51) compared to the general population in the United States (Average 1.61).

Prevalence of Adverse Childhood Experiences

ACE Score	CDC Study (N=17,337)	Camp HOPE Children (N=64)
0	36.1%	0.0%
1	26.0%	4.8%
2	15.9%	4.8%
3	9.5%	11.1%
4+	12.5%	79.4%

The Average Number of ACEs = 5.51

More importantly, we found that Camp HOPE has a significant positive impact on children exposed to domestic violence. A camp focused on increasing hope in the lives of children instead of focusing on reducing negative behaviors can reduce the impact of profound childhood trauma. We found significant increases in hope as reported by children a month before camp to the last night of camp. This increase in hope was sustained 30 days after camp. Finally, the findings demonstrated that children's self-reported hope was related to behaviors associated with positive character development. This means that if we can raise hope, we will see positive character development which can also mitigate trauma and empower children to set better goals for their lives. Raising hope is far less expensive and far more humane than simply spending more and more money locking up rage-filled children and adults for their crimes and abuse of others.

Camp HOPE America provides powerful evidence that rising hope can change the way children impacted by domestic violence, like Gemma, view themselves and their futures. It is one of many programs now being identified across the country that is increasing hope in the lives of children and teens that might otherwise end up in the prisons and mental health facilities of this country. The chart below demonstrates the measurable way that hope is increasing in children coming to camp each summer in a program where the science of hope is being applied.

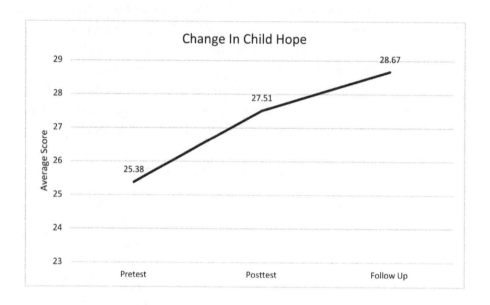

Children exposed to domestic violence live in chaos and fear. The pain of that chaos and fear produces rage, despair, and eventually apathy. Hope is a psychological strength that can mitigate that rage, despair, and apathy. It is a protective resource that can help children cope with stress and adversity associated with domestic violence as they are inspired to set goals and find pathways. Children with high levels of hope have a greater capacity to identify viable pathways and dedicate mental energy to their goals. In the absence of these positive strengths, victimization from and perpetration of violence are much more likely than in those with no ACEs-related trauma in their lives.

Gemma's story has been replicated hundreds of times now in our research. Our study demonstrated that hopeful children seek positive opportunities (zest, grit, optimism, curiosity), learn to better regulate thoughts and feelings (self-control), and can better understand and appreciate the actions, motives and feelings of others (social intelligence, gratitude). Rising hope does not solve all the challenges of healing from abuse but it helps children and adult survivors to begin the journey.

Lessons Learned from Abused Kids

After fourteen years of developing our special camp for children impacted by domestic violence, we have learned some lessons that will help everyone aspiring to see rising hope in their lives.

- **Everybody deserves and needs to be loved.** Children and adults with high ACE scores don't always know what real love is, and many don't believe they deserve to be loved. They mistake unhealthy attention for love. Children act out for attention, and adults can easily focus on the misconduct and miss the cry for love. They may not know how to express it, but it is there crying out through their anger, pain, and shame.

- **Call everyone in your life by their name.** It has always bothered both of us when people call children "buddy" or "sweetheart" or "kiddo," usually because they don't know their name. Even as adults, we know whether someone remembers our name because if they know it, they use it. Take time to learn a child's name. Take time to learn an adult's name and then call them by name. Names matter. If you don't remember someone's name, ask them, and then use his or her name in sentences and conversation until you remember it.

- **Caring conversation and active listening are hope-giving.** Many hurting people don't need fancy programs, a lot of gifts, and complex activities to begin to heal and find pathways to hope. They need to be listened to. They need to be asked what happened to them. Children and adults need a loving and caring person to ask good questions and listen to the answers. Caring conversation is where children can be challenged to think about goals, motivation, and pathways to their goals. You can talk to them about little daily goals or long-term bigger goals.

- **Children need to celebrate their childhood.** Children with trauma in their lives often grow up too fast. They have been forced to experience adult power and control. Or they had to take the role of the parent. When a child must handle certain emotions and experience psychological responses too young, they miss out on the pure joy of childhood. Next time you are tempted to say when a child is upset or crying over some struggle or pain in their life, "Just grow up," stop yourself. Shut your mouth. Hug and comfort them. And then think of a way you can help give them their childhood back.

- **Fun is therapeutic.** The therapeutic power of adventure, fun, laughter, joy, and freedom is measurable. They help increase hope in our lives. The next time a counselor asks you to sit in an office for an hour suggest a walk to the ice cream store. Suggest an hour of talking and bowling. Next time your underwear is all up in a wad and you think a child just really needs an intense talking to, try grabbing a Melatonin instead and proposing something fun with the child. You can talk if you need to while throwing a Frisbee or playing with the dog. You will be surprised how much better the "talk" will go.

- **We can all live without technology.** Children struggle to give their technology. Parents are glued to it even when out to eat with the family. Once you put it down, set a few other goals, and pursue them, you will be amazed how your senses come alive. After a few hours of fun or games or adventure without electronics, you are still alive and the universe is still in place. The earth keeps rotating around the sun. Try it.

- **Nature is therapeutic.** We have seen children find their sense of wonder again in nature at camp. Fascinated by the simplest sounds or smells, children and adults come alive in nature. For some, your idea of camping is the Hampton Inn and your idea of nature is a plastic plant in the corner of your office. But if you want rising hope, go spend some time in the beauty of the world around you.

- **Music, art, writing, and drama unleash creative, healing energy.** Silly songs around a campfire, even in your backyard, do wonders for a sad heart. Writing in a journal, drawing pictures of hope, kindness, courage, and compassion, and telling stories (made up or true) to others produce creativity and healing energy in the lives of human beings.

- **We all long for a sense of community and a culture of hope.** Children and adults love to belong to a group of people who care about each other. For years, after watching the TV show *"Cheers,"* we were pretty sure you could only find that in a bar. Turns out there are many more places to find community and feel hope. If you don't have a healthy extended family where you can find community, you need to create it somewhere else. We all need to belong and we all need to be around people with high hope.

- **We all need things to look forward to in life.** We saw early in Camp HOPE that one week of camp raised Hope scores, but one week was not enough. The kids needed things to look forward to all year long. It is why we have created a year-round Pathways to HOPE Program for abused children and we have proven that this allows their elevated Hope scores from camp to stay high all year long. But we all need that. Everyone wants things to look forward to in life. Without exciting goals in our future, we can get stuck in the now. Living in the present is great and enjoying what we are doing now is healthy. But if you want to stay healthy, make sure you have goals to look forward to in your life and pick pathways that can help make you make hope happen.

- **Gratitude is cathartic.** Grateful adults and children have higher hope than those who lack the ability to appreciate what they have or to appreciate others in their lives. Our findings mirror those of Brené Brown. Children with higher gratitude are more joyful as well. Gratitude increases hope and joy. We need to practice gratitude. It does not always come naturally. Put down this book and go thank someone for what they did for you. Decide to communicate gratitude and appreciation every day and teach your children how to do it as well. It will heal something in you and help raise your level of hope.

- **Some children and adults need professional help.** We have both been to counseling. We have both needed professional help to navigate our trauma. Let's work hard to reject the stigma that some might put on us for needing professional help. Rising hope helps brain development in a child. Goal setting and goal achievement can increase motivation for adults to move forward in life no matter what the obstacles they face. But sometimes we really need a counselor, a nutritionist, or a doctor to help us navigate in our lives. When somebody makes fun of you for doing what you need or looks sideways at you, call BS and then go make your next appointment.

- **Give children permission and space to explore spiritual truth.** The research is very clear that spiritual faith can play a powerful role in producing rising hope in the lives of trauma survivors. Many children impacted by trauma have never had loving, caring exposure to transparent, honest spirituality. Some children have even been abused or manipulated by those using religion or faith as tool of their abuse. Spiritual support ranks high in all the research on the needs of trauma survivors. We need to give children a pathway to find out how they can access a loving God.

The amazing children of Camp HOPE America, like Gemma, can teach us a few things about hope. They help us see that hope is not just an emotion. They help us see that talking about it and focusing on how to increase it can change the pathways of our lives—every one of us. It is also clear that if you are struggling to be the parent your children need, rising hope will give you the best chance to become that loving, supportive parent. Parents with low hope will rarely produce children with high hope. Parents with high hope will give their children the greatest chance of success in life. Gemma's mom also experienced abuse in her childhood and it has been hard for her to have Gemma talk about her pain from childhood. Gemma has had to learn to encourage her mother's goals and has helped her mother talk more about what she experienced as a child. We love to see young people becoming role models for their parents even if their parents struggle with lower levels of hope.

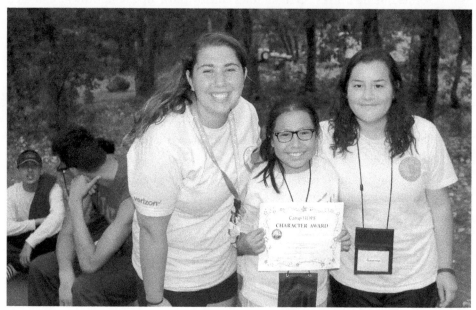

Gemma (right) at Camp HOPE America (2017)

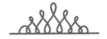

Chapter 13

Lessons Learned from Battered Women

"Once I felt like I was really in a community where I belonged, I didn't feel alone anymore. I didn't feel like my happiness in life depended on one person doing and saying the right thing to me on any given day. I don't know why I lived my life that way for so long. It was a terrible way to live. Imagine expecting one man to meet all my needs, every day, for my whole life. He can barely conjugate a sentence after getting home from work, let alone be everything I needed him to be. I am pretty sure I was doomed to expect that his anger and dysfunction was going to disappear the day we married. He blamed his shit on me, but it really was his shit."

—**Annabelle**, San Diego Family Justice Center Client

Lisbet

Lisbet came to the United States illegally with her husband. He was violent and abusive in their marriage right from the beginning. Her three children had to endure his violence and rage until he was finally deported after being arrested for domestic violence. Lisbet came to the San Diego Family Justice Center for help in 2009. At the Family Justice Center, she found 25 agencies all together under one roof and she found a community of support and encouragement. She found friends. She found other women with children who needed love and support just like she and her kids did. One of the Center's partners was a local shelter, Project Safehouse, run by a nonprofit called the Center for Community Solutions. Project Safehouse gave her a place to live with her kids. Two years later, other survivors at the Family Justice Center asked her to join a committee called VOICES to help them advocate for other victims and their kids in San Diego. She started telling her story publicly on television and to audiences throughout the community. As she shared her story, she found more friends with a similar story. A year after that, Lisbet's three children started attending Camp HOPE San Diego. Her children started finding their own hope hanging out with other children with similar experiences.

Lisbet was a high school graduate but had no other education. Employment prospects were slim for making a living that would support her family. But she decided to set a goal of owning her own business. Her family though knew the world of janitorial services as do many immigrants. In 2013, Alliance for HOPE International gave her a $3,000 micro-loan from the Verizon Foundation to help her start JCL Janitorial. She hired a few of her relatives and started building her business.

In 2014, Lisbet won the contract to have her company clean the very shelter, Project Safehouse, that she lived in with her kids in 2009 after fleeing from her abusive husband. Today, Lisbet still runs her janitorial business, advocates for other survivors in a program called Proyecto Esperanza (Project Hope), and is taking college classes to pursue a social work degree. The support of a community that welcomed her in, motivated her to set goals and provided real pathways for her to find her way to healing and a future. Her children too are finding their own goals and pathways—and rising Hope scores—in their participation in Camp HOPE America and our year-round mentoring activities. Lisbet needed what we all need—a community that she could belong to, not just a program or pity.

Domestic Violence Survivors

While the findings for Camp HOPE are amazing, we wanted to see if hope has similar protective factors for survivors of domestic violence receiving services at Family Justice Centers. Family Justice Centers, now operating in more than 40 states and 20 countries, are multi-disciplinary and multi-agency Centers where victims of domestic violence, sexual assault, elder abuse, human trafficking, and other forms of violence can come one place to get help. In so many situations today, without a Family Justice Center framework, victims must go from agency to agency and place to place, telling their story repeatedly. For many victims, the journey of receiving services at many locations is too burdensome and in the process, many lose hope and return to their abusive situations.

The Family Justice Center framework, promulgated by Alliance for HOPE International, seeks to create pathways to hope for survivors and their children, and the pathway often begins with one place they can go to get as many services as possible. In this model, professionals can work together and share information and resources—allowing for a community of support and advocacy that addresses a victim's needs in a host of areas from the criminal justice system, to civil legal help, to medical services, to mental health services and spiritual care, to job training, and other advocacy and support.

Victims of domestic violence are at an increased risk for anxiety, depression, social isolation, and substance use/abuse. It is estimated that 1 in 3 women will experience domestic violence in her lifetime. 1 in 5 women will experience sexual assault in their lifetime. The physical and psychological impact of domestic violence and sexual assault is a clear public health concern with a tremendous economic impact in the billions of dollars. Family Justice Centers offer a multi-disciplinary, single location for survivors and their children.

We have heard many stories about survivors finding their way to hope and healing like Lisbet. But could we prove that bringing all the professionals, volunteers, and community volunteers into one place would be the kind of culture of hope that would increase it in the lives of hurting families coming to these Centers for help?

Victims in focus groups that Casey and the CEO of Alliance for HOPE International, Gael Strack, have conducted for over a decade have been consistent in saying that they would like to be able to go one place instead of having to go from agency to agency, telling their story repeatedly. So, we knew victims had expressed their desire to come one place for help and support. But was greater "community" being created with professionals from multiple disciplines coming together under one roof? Blue Shield of California Foundation funded a study for us so we could answer these questions.

318 survivors completed hope assessments at the time of intake in California-based Centers and then again approximately 45-60 days later. We also measured their ACE scores. These survivors had an average ACE score of 3.31 with just under 50% having four or more adverse childhood experiences.

When we compared hope at intake to the 45-60 day follow up, survivors reported significant increases in their hope. These increases in survivor hope were related to higher life satisfaction, emotional well-being, and the capacity to flourish.

Finally, hope was a significant predictor of goal attainment for the survivors. If hope increased in the lives of survivors, we always found that they were more likely to be achieving their own goals. Like children from Camp HOPE, we found that hope is a significant protective factor for survivors of domestic violence. The chart below demonstrates the power of hope, using the science of hope in the lives of more than 318 survivors just like Lisbet.

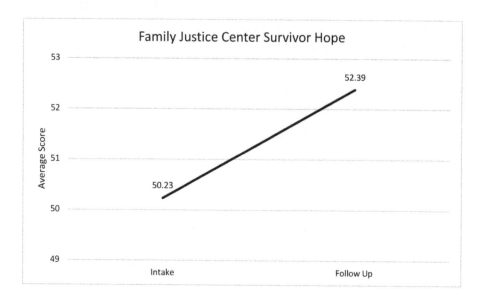

Hope Can Be Learned

One afternoon, Chan's two-year old grandson (Emerson) came to visit his office at the University. In one corner of the office, Chan has a few golf clubs, a basketball, tennis racquet and some tennis balls. When he saw these items, Emerson was motivated to play with these new toys. To reduce their stress, Emerson's parents placed his stroller in front of the clubs creating a barrier to his goal. While Emerson experienced a momentary frustration (emotion is an outcome of hope), his ability to find alternative pathways to get the toys helped reinforce that he had the power to achieve his future goal. As Emerson began to experience success by overcoming the barrier, his agency level was enhanced resulting in higher hope. This moment in time was a great opportunity for Emerson to practice hope by learning how to problem solve to achieve his desired goal (get the toys). The result of Emerson's rising hope? Chan's office was a mess.

Emerson's story highlights two key points. First, we can and do have opportunities to experience hope very intentionally every day. In Emerson's case, a small amount of adversity was useful in learning how to solve problems that will transfer to his ability to flourish in the future. The second key point is most important for all of us to understand—Hope can be learned.

Our research with Camp HOPE and the survivors getting help in Family Justice Centers provide empirical support that we can move the needle on hope. We are essentially teaching survivors (adults and children) how to move their own needle on hope through goal setting and goal achievement. Because hope is a cognitive process, we can learn new pathways to our goals on our own. We can learn how to solve problems to overcome barriers, strategize alternative workable pathways, or shift our goals to better align within the realm of what is possible. Sometimes, this process requires the support of others (i.e., friend, loved one, coach, teacher, counselor, etc.) who can help us appropriately frame our experiences and sometimes we can figure out most of it on our own.

With practice, we can also learn to regulate our mental energy. We can learn to focus our attention and willpower to our pathways. Just like Colette in her journey to hope that we saw earlier, Lisbet learned to narrow her focus early to how to make her business successful. She wanted to go to college right away after she left her abuser but first she needed to figure out how to provide for her family. Today, many years later she is using her mental energy to focus on becoming a college graduate.

Lessons Learned from Abused Women

In recent years, women and some men that have survived violence and abuse have interacted with us in many ways. Like the name of the advocacy group our survivors have created in Family Justice Centers, VOICES, they have used their voices to teach us some things about finding higher hope. Like Lisbet, they have shared some of the goals they have set for themselves. We have found in our research most of their goals can help all of us find rising hope.

- **Be nice to yourself**—So many women have talked about blaming themselves and being angry with themselves after their own poor choices or ending up in a bad situation. Then, they say how much it meant to them for someone at a Family Justice Center to offer them a cup of coffee, tea, the chance to go for a walk, some quiet time with a little soft music in a room alone. They have said they realized they needed to offer themselves those little kindnesses as well. Don't we all? Give yourself permission to take a few minutes right now for a little walk, some downtime, a little self-care. This type of centering helps with goal-setting as you clear your mind, change your scenery, or get a little exercise.

- **Shut out the bad stuff**—Colette did it. She turned off the news. Women in our survivor groups with rising Hope scores say that they stop reading the paper. Saturating your life with bombings, sexual harassment, rapes, wars, and scandals is detrimental to your long-term health. Some women and many couples have told us that when they stopped watching TV right before bedtime, they felt more restful and hopeful in the morning. This is a great strategy with your kids as well. In most of our research, when the kids get less negative messaging, they end up with higher hope.

- **Reject the negative self-talk**—Many survivors have told us that negative messaging inside their heads takes them to dark places often. We both have similar tapes playing in our heads at times. Brené Brown points out that sometimes our greatest critic is in the mirror. Our own negative self-talk rises in us and tells us we are not enough, we are not original, we don't have anything special to offer to the world, or we cannot succeed. We see it in the traumatized adults and children we support and study. "I'm not smart enough for college." "People like me don't get to do things like that." "I don't deserve to be happy after the things I have done." "I don't have the connections to get a job like that."

    Negative messaging from others or from inside your head will not create a pathway to hope. Most often, it is motivated by fear and you need to identify it and reframe it as an opportunity for courage in your life. Learning how to replace those messages with statements about your own capacity, giftedness, uniqueness, and abilities will help counteract the negative messaging. The American Psychological Association has said for years that you need 11 positive messages to overcome one negative message delivered to a child. It is true for adults as well. It is true for our own battles with the negative voices in our heads that so many of us live with every day. We need to surround ourselves with people that will believe in us, affirm us, encourage (put courage into us), and help rally us when we are down or when we fail at a goal. Negative messages most often damages our agency or motivation to pursue a goal. So, focusing on ways to increase our motivation is the antidote. Practicing positive self-talk is a great start.

- **Speak positive affirmations to yourself and others**—In abusive situations, both sides often get very hot. They see the other person as the problem and they make clear their views. Sometimes a violent or abusive person is the core problem. But many survivors have told us that as they learn more about the science, they meditate on statements like, "Peace in my life begins with me" or "I am the key to my own calm." For years, Casey and his family have sent out holiday greeting cards with the message, "Peace on Earth Begins at Home." Peace in your family begins in your home. Peace in your family often begins with peace in your heart and life. Try speaking those kinds of affirmations to yourself. "Peace in my life begins with my peace." "I am the key to peace in my life."

So many times, angry people think peace will come from how a social service agency helps them or some institution responds to the wrong they have experienced. In all our research, the opposite is true. Peace starts with an individual and it comes into the world only through peaceful individuals. We must learn to live it in our words and actions instead of giving in to fear, hatred, or resignation (apathy). Remember, resignation or apathy is the opposite of hope. Choosing to implement some of these actions (goals) has helped many survivors of trauma find hope and it will work whether you have ever been abused by another person or not.

- **Get close to people with high hope**—Many survivors tell us that their hope levels went up as soon as they started spending more time with higher hope friends. People with goals, motivation, and strategic thinking about their pathways are contagious. Oprah Winfrey puts it this way, "Surround yourself only with people who are going to lift you higher." We will always do better in life if we hang out with people with higher hope. People with lower hope pull us down and even if we work with them, are married to them, or live next door to them—we cannot spend all our time there. We need people with high hope around us.

- **Create a meditation/prayer time (3-5 Minutes)**—Women often talk to us about their need for prayer or meditation. You don't have to believe in God to make this work. Just light a candle and reflect quietly in a quiet place. Sometimes being outside helps with the breeze gently blowing on your face. Sometimes a room alone inside your house is better. When you first start, three minutes will seem like an eternity. Stick with it. You can get to five minutes as you develop a discipline. Practice your breathing—slow and consistent. Deep breaths. Hold them. Let them out slowly. Let them out slower than you took them in. A silence ritual like this can be powerful and centering for anyone. Many with profound trauma and even crisis often tell us this helps them think more clearly about goals and pathways. We dare you. Go do 3-5 minutes right now and then come back and keep reading. How does it feel? Did it feel like rising hope? Bet it did. Or you just kept reading and didn't invest the 3-5 minutes we just gave you.

- **Celebrate each day with gratitude**—We have seen in our research how much gratitude correlates to hope. Thankful people are more hopeful than entitled people who never appreciate the precious gift of life or kindness from others. Survivors that articulate a sense of appreciation for the support they receive or the help they are given have higher hope in their lives. A high Hope score connects directly to higher gratitude in someone's life. Be on the lookout every day for things and people that you can appreciate and look for ways to express it. Make a list of who you appreciate and why. Drop those folks a text message, note, or email. It will be positive in their lives AND in yours.

- **Look at the sky or feel the sun on your face**— Many battered women have expressed the bigness of the world and the importance of being in nature in their recovery journeys. Many Family Justice Centers, social service programs, and even mental health facilities are realizing that doing everything indoors is a bad idea. The sun, the moon, the stars, and the sky can be a touchstone for hope. Look up at the sky often. See the planes going by and reflect on how fast everyone moves and think about how nice it is to slow down and reflect. As we travel the country talking about hope, we more and more realize the need to sit in our backyards or go to a park and then we look up and reflect. We are all people in need of hope. Sometimes when we take the time to look up at the sky it helps us remember that.

- **Pour out healthy affection like water**—Never forget the importance of human touch and healthy affection for both children and adults. This does not mean you express physical touch when unwanted or unasked for! Many Hollywood producers, business leaders, and political leaders are losing their reputations and their jobs today because of their entitled, sexually oriented personal conduct. But hugs, words, notes, and acts of kindness are all ways to express love in tangible ways to those around us. Hug and kiss your children and grandchildren. When someone is kind, tell them. Leave small notes expressing gratitude often. The Bible's adage that "love covers a multitude of sins" relates to this. Expressing kindness and healthy affection is physically and emotionally comforting to the giver and the receiver of each loving act. You will notice their faults less. Sometimes just a touch to the arm of someone you are talking to can increase hope in both your lives.

- **Learn to re-goal**—Many survivors have shared with us how they had to change their goals to move forward. Many victims of unhealthy relationships want to fix the relationship. Their goal is to stay with their partner and be safe and healthy. But they cannot change their partners or make those they love do the work necessary to heal and change. They must then decide to be safe without their partners, find new relationships, and re-adjust their goals. This process of "re-goaling" is constant in those with higher hope. They regularly ask if a goal is still important to them or if the obstacles can be overcome. If they cannot be overcome, they choose to adjust their goals or pick new goals.

- **Go make a difference in another's life**—We teach adult and child survivors of abuse that hope is believing in yourself, believing in others, and believing in your dreams. If you spend all your time believing only in yourself and your own dreams, you become a narcissist. Each time you make a difference in someone else's life, you create hope in your own life. Serving others ends up being self-serving. Serving others serves up hope in your own life and in theirs. Survivors of abuse have told us over and over that when they get to help others, they feel better about themselves. Why? Hope is rising when you do that—add a little kindness to someone else's world. It is true for adults and true for kids. You can do too much for others and not refill your own tank and end up low in hope. But much of the time, we are not doing enough for others and no matter how much shopping, golf, or entertainment we pursue in our own lives, we still feel low hope. Try spending time doing something every week for others. It will produce a result in your life: Hope rising.

- **Practice movement daily**—There is overwhelming research coming out that there is a strong brain-body connection with trauma. Trauma changes the body and gets trapped inside you. This is true in adults and children. We have seen over and over that physically active survivors of abuse do better than those that are sedentary or rely only on counseling in an office to help them find their way forward. Bessel van der Kolk, Peter Levine, Linda Chamberlain and many others are finding that intentional movement and exercise promotes healing. Yoga is not the only effective brain-body modality that does this but it is a great example. We will talk about this more later.

How can it be that people with so much pain in their lives often have higher Hope scores than those with so much good in their lives—good jobs, benefits, material

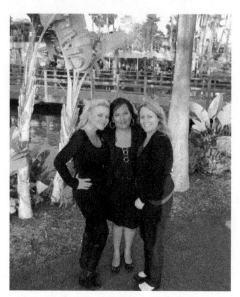

Lisbet (middle) with VOICES Members Kimberly and Yvonne

possessions, and little trauma? How can it be that the "hurting people" can teach us lessons about hope?

The research findings provide convincing evidence that trauma survivors that choose hope find a protective and empowering force in their lives. Once they find hope, they have powerful messages to deliver to all of us whether we have major trauma in our lives or not. Lisbet and her friends, pictured here, Kimberly and Yvonne, are now advocating for other survivors of violence and abuse through their advocacy group called VOICES. Other survivors are finding pathways forward, motivated and inspired by the rising hope of women like Lisbet, Kimberly, and Yvonne.

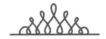

Chapter 14

Hope and the Human Brain

"What is my first memory in life? The day my Mom died."
—Lila, Age 14

Lila

Lila came to the San Diego Family Justice Center seven years ago with her mom. Her dad was in jail for domestic violence. Her mom Jillian seemed together at first. She was a nurse at a local hospital in San Diego. Jillian came to the Center to get a restraining order and counseling for herself. Lila was 10 years old at the time. She loved to read and quickly positioned herself in a bean bag chair in the corner of the children's room at the Center and began reading a book to her little sister, Darla, and her younger brother, Frank. It quickly became clear that Frank was on the autism spectrum, and struggled to concentrate as Lila read to them. The staff noticed quickly that Lila was responsible and mature. Not uncommon in abusive families, Lila had taken on the role of caretaker for her siblings. Lila presented as being so mature and articulate that staff members at the Center missed her needs. Jillian was very unstable and in desperate need of advocacy, legal services, and mental health assistance. Jillian was struggling to keep her job in the middle of an abusive relationship and could not provide for her children without it. The Family Justice Center staff offered counseling to Darla and Frank, but Jillian said she was just too busy to bring them in for separate counseling appointments that didn't coincide with her own, which took place while the kids were in school.

Lila, Darla, and Frank all signed up for Camp HOPE America that spring and came to camp for the first time that summer. At camp, the staff struggled to get Lila to participate in activities because she was a voracious reader and preferred a bench under a shady tree with a book in hand to any of the high adventure activities at camp. Three years passed as Jillian completed counseling and re-focused on work. Her kids kept coming to camp each summer, but Jillian never seemed to have the time to bring them in for counseling.

One fall day when Lila was 14, it became clear we had missed her complex needs. Lila's mom called the Center to tell them Lila was in the hospital and she wanted everyone to pray for her daughter. Lila had attempted suicide by slitting her wrists. Her mom confided that Lila was a "cutter" and this was not the first time it had happened—just the worst time. The Camp HOPE team had never seen her arms. Lila always wore long sleeves at camp.

Lila had to be put in a psychiatric lock-up unit at Rady Children's Hospital in San Diego while they tried to provide the help she needed. Two weeks into her treatment, Lila's psychiatrist asked her a question. "Lila, what is your first memory on your life?" Lila, slowly, quietly responded. "What is my first memory in life? The day my mom died." The psychiatrist was puzzled. Lila's mom, Jillian, was very much alive. As Jillian became involved in the follow up processing of Lila's disclosure, the truth emerged. Lila was only 2 ½ years old when Jillian was pregnant with Lila's brother, Frank. During that pregnancy, Jillian was beaten and strangled to the point of unconsciousness by her husband. Jillian did not know it, but Lila must have witnessed the assault and thought her mom was dead. This was Lila's first memory in life—buried in the recesses of her brain. It had never been disclosed, discussed, or addressed. Lila's brother was later born and diagnosed with autism. Jillian would go on to leave that abusive relationship and become a single parent. Lila would face profound, almost life-ending consequences from the memories burned deep into her subconscious.

Hope is a miracle of the human mind. Humans, alone, can be hopeful and future-oriented. Animals cannot. Shane Lopez analyzed the Gallup World Poll in 2013 and concluded that most people, regardless of age, have an optimistic bias— that is, believing that tomorrow holds some promise and that things can change for the better. Unlike other animals, homo sapiens alone developed self-awareness, imagination, and the ability to symbolically represent thoughts and experiences. Some attribute this to evolutionary processes alone. We attribute it to a Creator and

Master Designer. However you place yourself in the universe, by random chance or by divine appointment, our combination of imagination and time sensitivity gives us all the ability to think about the past and the future. We can stock up on meat and put it in a freezer in the garage. We can buy enough toiletries at Costco to last a year. We can remember the last time we ran out of gas and decide to fill up at a quarter of a tank. Our ability to anticipate future needs and plan accordingly makes us completely different than animals. What is the difference? Hope. Human beings have the capacity to hope.

Some believe hope comes from the brain, some believe it comes from the heart, and some believe it comes from the sacred and holy part of created beings. Shane Lopez often spoke to groups and challenged them to use his "Brain-Heart-Sacred Test." Most groups would split on their view of the part of human beings where hope finds its home. We tend to think the answer is all three. There is a brain part, there is a passion part, and there is a sacred and unexplainable part that sustains someone through pain, heartbreak, and even death.

The neurobiology of hope, however, is clearly an important piece of the puzzle. And there are enemies of hope like Lila experienced and we talked about in the discussion about ACEs. We will look more at enemies shortly but let's look at the neurobiology of hope because it helps explain how it works and how our ability to hope can be damaged by traumatic events like ACEs, other types of trauma, health and nutrition issues, or the daily stresses of life.

The Hope Engine of the Human Body—The Brain

Find a comfortable chair in a quiet place. Turn off the TV. Shut down your phone or computer. Finish reading the next paragraph and then go follow the directions below.

Close your eyes. Take a few deep breaths. Hold the breath in and then let it out slowly. Again. Let go of the worries of the day. Erase your mental to-do list. Lift your shoulders and then relax them. Are you ready? Now, imagine your life in five years. Pick a goal you want to pursue, think about the pathways to get there, and then envision yourself there. Maybe it is a new job, a new relationship, a healthier marriage, a new home, a disease-free body, the greatest vacation of your life, or something else that makes your heart happy. Pick just one. Are you ready? Go there now. Transport yourself into the future to the achievement of your goal. Five years have passed as you have now arrived in the future. Your future. You have arrived at this new place in your life. The goal is achieved. You found the pathways and you accomplished what you wanted to do or be. So, what do you see? What do you feel? What has changed in your life? Look around in your mind's eye. What does your future look like now that you are in it? Soak it in. What is happening around you? Who is there with you? As you get up and walk around, what is different? Why are you so happy? Why do you feel so much joy in your heart?

Now, let's talk about what just happened in this visioning exercise if you did it. You took memories from your past and then used them as the basis to begin to see the future. You processed what choices you need to make to get there. You thought about who else might be part of your goal and what it would feel like to accomplish it. You likely saw others with you five years from now—maybe people currently in your life and maybe new people that you created in your mind from a composite of people you have already known or seen. You could feel the emotions of attaining your goal in the future. You could feel joy, happiness, serenity, achievement, pride, and a sense of accomplishment. You could think about the steps you took to get there. You may have even felt the motivation that would be necessary for your goal to become reality.

What was happening during this visioning exercise? How was your brain functioning? If it was difficult for you to do the exercise, what reasons might explain the challenge of the exercise being successful? The answers to these are all about the neurobiology of hope.

Let's take a quick tour of the brain and use it to deconstruct our visioning exercise.

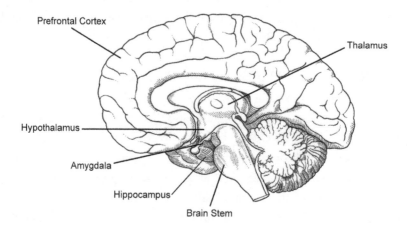

The Prefrontal Cortex—The command center of the brain and the planner of your future. This is where hope lives and where you figure out pathways to the future.

The Limbic System—The older part of the brain where instincts and natural reactions to stimuli occur including the activities of your hippocampus (the memory center), thalamus (the sensory center), and the amygdala (the fear center). Let's look at each part of the Limbic System.

- Hippocampus—This is where memories are formed and organized and it is also the brain's simulator where you mentally practice for the future.
- Thalamus—This is the sensory center of the brain (sight, sound, smell, touch, taste) that translates what you experience and sends messages to the other parts of the brain.
- Hypothalamus—The hypothalamus is mainly responsible for motivational behavior. It is the reason we know when we are hungry or thirsty. The hypothalamus helps our body maintain a constant temperature. It also controls the *pituitary gland*, which is the master gland that controls most of the release of hormones and other chemicals (including your adrenal glands) in a variety of circumstances to regulate body functions as needed.
- Amygdala—This is where you decide if you are threatened or in danger. It operates as an instinctual trigger urging you to seek safety when you are in danger. This is the home of your body's fight-flight-freeze response, which is often instinctual and is not always something you can control in a life-threatening or dangerous situation.

The Brain Stem (at the bottom of the diagram)—The oldest part of the brain, sometimes referred to as the reptilian brain, maintains involuntary blood circulation and respiratory function

Deconstructing the Visioning Exercise

Your prefrontal cortex processed our request to sit down, relax, and stretch. Once you started thinking about your goal—small or large—you began using your hippocampus to process past goals and experiences that related to your goal. The amygdala stayed calm in the process and helped you keep a future orientation in the absence of a scary or life-threatening vision of your future. The chemicals that your HPA axis (Hypothalamic-Pituitary-Adrenal) might otherwise have released to deal with a high energy, challenging, or scary situation were dormant and this allowed your hippocampus to do its job without interruption—helping you process memories and then allowing your pre-frontal cortex to turn them into dreams for your future. This is the neurobiology of hope at work. But what happens when things go wrong?

What happens when the fear is real? What happens when your ACEs through childhood mess up the way your brain is supposed to operate? What happens when the hope engine stops working right? Lila's hope engine was badly damaged when she was so very little and it has not fully recovered. Her mother's brain may well have suffered a traumatic brain injury (TBI) from being strangled or hit in the head as many victims do experience. How can we understand better what happened to Lila's hope engine and why it is so hard now for her to think about the future and imagine a special future for herself?

When Fear Moves In, And Doesn't Leave

For many, fear is simply an emotion, the most universal and often most painful emotion. But there is much more to understand about fear. Dr. David Lisak says fear is at the core of trauma. When fear is healthy, it reminds us of our limits as human beings. We get in dangerous situations and the amygdala fires and starts flashing danger signs to the pre-frontal cortex even as it starts pumping cortisol and corticosteroids to help us respond as needed to protect ourselves. When facing the worst of threats, it produces the strength for a man to lift a car off his wife's body after a tragic accident. We become real life super heroes for brief, lifesaving moments. The amygdala masks our feeling of pain in our body when we are bleeding but still need to act to save our children from a dangerous situation. What happens? Blood vessels constrict, reducing trauma-induced blood loss, so we can protect those we love. Anti-inflammatory cortisol floods our bloodstream to temporarily quiet our pain so that we can act. Healthy fear sees a threat and our brain warns us to change course or take evasive action. Security expert Gavin de Becker focuses on intuition in threat situations saying "…intuition is always right in at least two important ways; It is always in response to something. It always has your best interest at heart." But our stress response can get stuck in overdrive.

Toxic Stress

The Center on the Developing Child at Harvard University has looked closely at toxic stress in children. As we have seen, when a child is threatened, the body responds automatically by increasing heart rate, blood pressure, and stress hormones (like cortisol). The body returns fairly quickly to the baseline we saw at the beginning of this chapter if the child is living in a safe environment and has strong supportive parents, friends, and family. But if the stress response gets stuck in overdrive, damage can begin to happen. The longer the stress response is extreme it begins to weaken the human body, damage brain architecture in children and adults, and can produce lifelong impacts as we saw in the ACE study.

The Harvard team has identified and defined each type of stress response:

Positive stress response—is a normal part of everyday life when there are brief increases in heart rate and mild increases in hormone levels in children, for example, when they go to a dentist for the first time or enter a new school;

Tolerable stress response—occurs when the body experiences something scary or frightening. We have touched on this related to a hurricane or forest fire or being injured or terrified about something. If it does not last long and there are supportive parents, friends, and family members after the child goes through the experience, the brain and body recover fairly quickly;

Toxic stress response—occurs when a child or adult experiences something that is not brief, but is prolonged or frequent. We have seen these types of situations throughout the book related to physical, sexual, or emotional abuse, bullying, community violence, chronic neglect, or children having to navigate life all alone like part of Chan's story we shared at the beginning of the book. This kind of prolonged activation can disrupt brain development in a child, can impact organ systems, and increase the risk of stress-related disease or other kinds of cognitive impairment. It can then play itself out throughout adulthood.

The good news is that rising hope, which includes supportive relationships, goal setting, and critical thinking to find pathways to goal achievement can prevent or reverse the damaging impacts of toxic stress response.

But, without intervention, the stress-activated fear response can take us off course from our goals and dreams—in a high-pitched screaming force in our brains called hypervigilance.

Hypervigilance

Hypervigilance is a state of hyper-arousal that usually connects to PTSD as we talked about in our discussion of ACEs. Hypervigilance sometimes develops in those with major recurring trauma who end up in a constant state of tenseness as the brain essentially gets stuck in high alert. Dr. Nadine Burke Harris, in *The Deepest Well*, describes it as a normal, short-term state when we are in the woods running from a bear. But it becomes destructive in the context of a soldier living in a combat zone every day, refugees fleeing for their lives from civil war, a family living in a gang-infested neighborhood where every day there is fear and many nights there are gunshots, or abused children who are living with their abuser every day. Going back to the forest metaphor, it is always being afraid of a bear in the woods even when there is no bear.

We see fear and its byproduct, hypervigilance, often in our research around hope, particularly when measuring trauma exposure in adults or children. When we talk about trauma, we are fundamentally talking about fear. It manifests itself when we see a child at camp scanning the environment moment by moment for potential threats. We see it in battered women in shelters when they fear their abuser will show up at any moment even in the safety of a locked facility. We have seen it in refugee populations in the Middle East or in new immigrants to the United States. People displaying hypervigilance often ignore close friends or family members in favor of the scrutiny of their surroundings that they must employ moment by moment. They tend to overreact to loud bangs or unexpected noises. Crowds will often make them agitated or too much noise. A person's body language may trigger them or a change in voice or tone—all of which are being constantly assessed in a person living with hypervigilance.

Years ago, in our first camping projects with abused kids, we allowed moms to come to camp with their children for a pilot program. What we did not know is that the children of the invited moms had all been sexually abused. The moms were hypervigilant and fearful of every counselor and staff member—suspecting them of molesting their children even during the most innocent of activities. Some of the fear-based reactions of the hypervigilant include:

- Lack of objectivity—reading too much into situations
- An over awareness of what people see or think about them
- Looking for others to betray them constantly
- Constantly concerned about others
- Not being aware of what is obvious to others
- Over scrutinizing/analyzing behavior of situations

Fear-based reactions are often normal reactions to abnormal experiences in life. But such a chronic, toxic stress state, as we have seen, can be damaging physiologically and emotionally.

Living in fear can suck hope right out of our lives. Author Max Lucado describes it this way: "[Fear] sucks the life out of the soul, curls us into an embryonic state, and drains us dry of contentment. We become abandoned barns, rickety and tilting from the winds, a place where humanity used to eat, thrive, and find warmth. No longer. When fear shapes our lives, safety becomes our god. When safety becomes our god, we worship the risk-free life. Can the safety lover do anything great? Can the risk averse accomplish noble deeds? For God? For others? No. The fear-filled cannot love deeply. Love is risky. They cannot give to the poor. Benevolence has no guarantee of return. The fear-filled cannot dream wildly. What if their dreams sputter and fall from the sky? The worship of safety emasculates greatness."

We need to face fear in the journey of choosing hope. But there is also another low-grade form of fear that often invades the lives of those with low levels of hope. It is called anxiety.

Anxiety

Tricia

Tricia lives with panic attacks. They come upon her suddenly and without warning. A touch of a stranger might trigger one. A smell might send her into almost a catatonic state. Sometimes they are short and sometimes she will come out of one and find hours have passed. She has ended up on the ground unable to get up, frozen in place in a car (called tonic immobility), or even lying in bed unable to move. Her doctors have tried medication but she becomes a zombie and can hardly function in day to day life. She lives with a sense of dread when they will come and how long they will last. Tricia has been often startled by unexpected, loud sounds and is embarrassed to talk about them with even close friends.

As they have haunted her over the years, her panic attacks have gotten worse. Depression has crept in, impacting her relationship with her children and her husband. Her husband tired of them over the years and the lack of empathy and support eventually led them to divorce. Separation and divorce though didn't end the all-consuming moments and sometimes hours when she found herself paralyzed with fear and anxiety from things she did not understand and could not seem to control. Years later, a therapist would help her unlock past experiences that had sent her slowly down the descent into crippling fear, chronic anxiety, and then uncontrollable panic attacks. Today, she is slowly finding herself and her way back to normal days and healthy relationship with a great deal of professional help. It is not an easy process.

Anxiety is born and nurtured in fear. It too does damage to hope. It is not as easy to see as abject terror or amygdala-firing fear. Max Lucado has called anxiety a "cold wind that won't stop howling in our minds." We struggle to relax. We cannot let our guard down. Every time we feel peaceful, it is only a brief interruption from the constant buzz of "what ifs" that rain down on us almost all the time. Many live with it every day in this country.

The National Institute of Mental health says that anxiety disorders are at an all-time high in the United States. How many people struggle with anxiety—low grade fear—at one time or another each year? More than 49 million Americans will experience at least one phobia, anxiety disorder, or panic attack. And it gets worse. According to the World Health Organization, nearly one-third of all Americans will suffer from an anxiety disorder in their lifetime.

Most of us know the feeling—a churning stomach, a sense of foreboding, difficulty breathing at the thought of certain events happening in our lives, a lack of control over our lives that feels paralyzing. Anxiety and fear are related, but not the same. Fear usually means there is a real threat. Anxiety conjures up imaginable threats. Fear is only a healthy emotion if we really need one of its three options: fight, flight, or freeze.

We have seen how anger or rage is an imposter of hope. Frustration and anger simply tell us that our goals have not been met, our expectations are not matching our lived experience. Fear cannot get us to hope either. The fear signals when you are in a dangerous situation trigger a whole-body response that gives us the resources to quite literally fight, run, or "play dead." Our friend Gavin de Becker called it "the gift of fear" many years ago. Our primal instinct is to sense danger. Gavin posited that, for many people, when bad things happened, they had ignored those instincts. The woman walking to her apartment door that sensed she was being followed and ignored the feeling until the man was pushing his way in her front door. The man who senses he is too close to the edge of the cliff but ignores the fear center of his brain sending warnings and falls off the cliff. When fear does its job, we often can avoid the potential harm that comes from what scares us. But we cannot live in a fear state all the time.

When the amygdala fires all the time, it is exhausting and produces a host of negative physical and emotional consequences. We saw the consequences in the research around the ACE Study and our discussion of the potential impacts on the developing brain in a child or young person.

But we must be aware of anxiety as well. Anxiety doesn't come from the fight-flight-freeze response. Anxiety comes from uneasiness with our circumstances or discouragement from our inability to see positive pathways forward in life. Anxiety comes when the lack of positive pathways turns into dread and a sense of doom. Anxiety and its common companion, stress, produce terrible consequences in our lives. Anxiety does not pump us up for a great day, put a spring in our step, or give us a greater sense of control over our lives. We all know the high cost that fear and anxiety produce in our daily lives. No one ever got healthier by living in more fear. No one ever found that embracing their fears or phobias made them a better parent or partner. Nobody ever says, "I just needed to spend more time living every day with anxiety, and my immune disorder started to subside." Tricia had to learn to face her fears and address not only the screaming dangers in her panicked moments but the low-grade quiet threat—fear's cousin anxiety—that she lived with between the panic attacks. We see it as all connected to low hope.

Is Anxiety Simply the Failed Pursuit of Happiness?

British author Ruth Whippman in her book, *America the Anxious: How Our Pursuit of Happiness is Creating a Nation of Nervous Wrecks*, doesn't blame anxiety on low hope. She argues that our anxiety comes from our relentless pursuit of happiness—an elusive and unattainable goal for most of us.

As a cynic of American culture, Whippman mocks mindfulness and a host of other pathways that people shared with her in the pursuit of their goal of happiness. "Their answers range from the mundane to the mind boggling. Yoga and meditation. Keeping a 'gratitude journal.' A weekend seminar to Unleash the Power Within. Keeping your baby attached to your body for a minimum of twenty-two hours out of every twenty-four, and, most bafflingly, not least on a practical level, the drinking of wolf colostrum. A friend of a friend that I meet for coffee livens up a rather dull conversation about what time her husband gets home from work with the observation that it really doesn't matter one way or the other, as the most important person in her life is actually Jesus." Whippman ignores the research behind practices like yoga, meditation, spirituality, and mindfulness—all of which decrease anxiety and stress and increase calm and peace. But her criticism of the pursuit of happiness is a fair criticism of the American psyche.

Whippman continues: "The whole process starts to become painfully, comically neurotic. Work day contentment starts to give way to a low-grade sense of inadequacy when pitched against capital-H Happiness. The goal is so elusive and hard to define, it's impossible to pin point when it's even been reached, a recipe for anxiety." Her critique of American culture and the pursuit of happiness makes an excellent point of how certain goal selection in our lives may well increase anxiety rather than produce the desired goal attainment.

We don't agree with Ruth Whippman. The genesis of anxiety is low hope. It may be a result of pursuing unhealthy goals or unattainable goals. It may be the result of chronic fear from childhood taking up residence in our daily lives. But either way, it comes back to low hope—usually focused on our lack of power and control over large portions of our lives.

Choose Hope, Not Happiness, To Move Away from Fear and Anxiety

Our premise is not that Americans should work harder at being happy. The likely problem in America and with many others suffering from high rates of anxiety around the world is that we have low Hope scores either because we are pursuing unrealistic or unfulfilling goals or because we don't have the pathways to achieve the ephemeral goal of happiness. The research tends to point to hope as at least a symptom of happiness and most likely a pathway to greater happiness. The question becomes: Is it better to pursue rising hope or to pursue greater happiness? Hope preserves well-being when faced with the negative events of life. Those with higher hope have less anxiety than those with lower hope. Higher hope people, therefore, suffer less effects from negative life events and are often shielded from the impacts of adversity, they are better protected from the degrading power of stress and sadness—likely making room for more happiness.

Dr. Shane Lopez cited a study in *Making Hope Happen* that found that firefighters with higher hope coped with the natural day to day stresses of their job better, suffered less vicarious trauma and, therefore, were better able to avoid damaging stress than were firefighters with low Hope scores. Researchers concluded that with less anxiety to manage (from the impacts of stress at work), we are able to enjoy happier lives.

Since 1972, research in the United States has remained constant in polling—about 30% of Americans report they are "very happy." Hundreds of self-help books, mindfulness initiatives, megachurches, and thousands of life coaches have failed to change that number. Choosing to pursue hope is likely a better path to happiness and contentment than choosing to pursue happiness in and of itself.

As we saw in the neurobiology of hope earlier, when you are living daily with an amygdala in constant overdrive, you are not able to choose hope. You end up living for far too long in what we called earlier the survival window—the period of time when you cannot focus on hope in the middle of trauma or a major life-threatening situation. The decision-making around goal setting and pathways that opens the door is in your pre-frontal cortex. The pre-frontal cortex is where you conduct the executive functions needed to convert vision to reality. When we are using the pre-frontal cortex, we can connect ourselves to the future by way of a goal that matters to us. When fear drives our lives, day in and day out, we are not able to use our pre-frontal cortex to create goals, build relationships that sustain our motivation, and critically think about pathways to achieve our goals.

Traumatic Brain Injury

Traumatic brain injury (TBI) has been defined as "an alteration in brain function, or other evidence of brain pathology, caused by an external force," that may cause cognitive impairment. The numbers of those who experience TBI are not small. It is estimated that 1.5—2 million people experience a TBI each year. Many never even seek medical attention and experience short or long-term side effects without any treatment. We touch on it here because it can certainly impact a person's ability to set goals, find motivation, and identify pathways to goal achievement. Recent research has identified high rates of TBI in battered women, abused children, athletes, military personnel, and car accident victims.

Multiple TBIs become particularly dangerous and are cumulative. This is the type of situation that is causing chronic traumatic encephalopathy (CTE), that has been diagnosed in boxers, soccer players, MMA fighters, NFL football players, and battered women. TBIs and their treatment are complex but it is important to be aware of conditions that TBIs can cause such as depression, suicidality, CTE, and Alzheimer's-like syndromes. With the high numbers of TBIs, there are many that may need medical treatment and support to help mitigate the impacts as much as possible. Some readers may need far more medical and mental health assistance if you have suffered one or more TBIs. Medical treatment may be necessary before some can focus on hope. Mind-body strategies are particularly important for opening the door to hope after trauma, abuse, TBIs, or other adversity in life.

Embrace the Power of Mind-Body Strategies

There is tremendous work being done in the trauma recovery research world that focuses on ways to release trauma and anxiety from the body. When adults or children are "stuck" in fear, anxiety, hypervigilance, or other internalized impacts from a loss of control in their lives, hope fades and the attendant consequences are not good. From a scientific and physiological standpoint, the body can get stuck in a sympathetic state (fight, flight, or freeze response). The domino effect that ensues causes all kinds of hormonal and physical impacts.

Children and adults exposed to trauma often have difficulty focusing or paying attention. This inability to focus connects directly to difficulties in goal-setting and goal pursuit required in the science of hope. An all too common result in children with an inability to focus is a diagnosis of Attention Deficit Hyperactivity Disorder (ADHD) or Affective Disorders (depression, bipolar, or anxiety). Within allopathic medical spheres, the preferred answer is medication. It is big business. Last year, we spent $16.1 billion in this country to drug children with these types of diagnoses. Sadly, many children are being misdiagnosed and given anti-psychotic drugs that have their own long-term consequences. One consequence of these drugs is that they block the production of dopamine, which is so important for a child's motivation in life. While medication may be necessary for some, a growing body of research shows that movement and exercise are a less expensive alternative with little or no side effects. Brain-body activities can help produce dopamine, release trauma, and help children self-regulate more effectively. Let's look more closely at what the research is pointing toward around self-regulation and brain-body strategies and research.

Dr. Peter Levine has developed a technique called Somatic Experiencing. It involves working with a specially trained therapist to re-connect to sensations in your body to relieve the symptoms of PTSD. Somatic therapy is based on the theory that trauma symptoms are the effects of instability of the autonomic nervous system (ANS) such as blood flow, breathing, and digestion. Somatic techniques are often used with other types of body movement, dance, or yoga in order to regulate the ANS and return it to a state of equilibrium and homeostasis.

Dr. Linda Chamberlain, a child trauma therapist, has been doing research on brain-body modalities to treat trauma in abused children for many years. Linda Chamberlain puts it this way: "A convergence of science, practice, and culture has helped us to recognize the key role of mind-body strategies in promoting resilience and healing trauma. From a neurobiological standpoint, it has become clear that we need interventions that engage the more primitive, survival area of the brain to address how trauma is stored in the body."

Linda Chamberlain's work has found that anxiety has an immediate impact on the way we breathe, which becomes part of a physiological cascade of the body's response to stress. In the same way, breathing can be utilized to help tame the nervous system and move back toward a parasympathetic response (the relaxation state). Children and adults need simple tools to deal with the predictable effects of dysregulation associated with trauma. Often combined with movement, breath work is so quick and easy to learn that these strategies are being taught to children as young as preschoolers. She has found that intentional movement, coupled with breathing exercises, produces impressive results. Take a moment to think about it. The breathing changes that take place when we experience stress cause a domino effect that can produce more stress. If we learn, as Dr. Chamberlain teaches, how to control breathing when we are met with stress or trauma, the domino effect can completely change. Breathing is one of several pathways toward changing our response to stress and, therefore, altering its physical manifestations. Educating children to become aware of body sensations and then teaching them how to regulate those sensations produces healing. If you are interested in more information to that end, Dr. Chamberlain helps manage a website on best practices for children exposed to domestic violence (www.promisingfutureswithoutviolence.org) that is a tremendous resource to many now working in the field.

Science is catching up with what many cultures have understood for generations about the instinct of the body to heal and the capacity of our brains to rewire and heal. Movement, whether we think of the longstanding tradition of soothing an infant by rocking, taking a walk to de-stress, or indigenous traditions of dance, has been an instinctual part of human history. In his latest book, *The Brain's Way of Healing*, Dr. Norman Doidge includes several chapters on mind-body practices including Feldenkrais, an awareness of movement modality that was developed in Israel after World War II. Feldenkrais employs movement strategies to improve posture, flexibility, coordination, athletic and artistic ability, as well as to help those with restricted movement, chronic pain and tension, neurological, development, and mental health issues.

Organizations like Capacitar International (www.capacitar.org) have been doing cross-cultural work to share mind-body-spirit practices around the globe for decades. Dr. Chamberlain and others are now using many of Capacitar's practices including Tai Chi, mindfulness, visualization, Pal Dan Gum movements, breath work, and Emotional Freedom Technique (EFT or "tapping") in schools, domestic violence shelters, batterers' intervention groups, adolescent peer educator programs, health clinics, hospitals and many other settings.

In a recent qualitative research project in domestic violence shelters in Finland, Linda Chamberlain found histories of polyvictimization in many of the victims (i.e. childhood trauma *and* adult domestic violence). Mind-body practices were found to be extremely beneficial in reducing the impacts of trauma with clients. On-site therapists and other staff confirmed the need of adults and children for self-calming and self-regulation. Mind-body practices are an essential part of the pathway to engaging effectively in services and healing. They also help open the door to higher hope— through better goal-setting and pathways thinking

Self-Regulation Comes First

Bessel van der Kolk argues that most effective treatments for trauma include four key steps related to the mind-body connection. First, self-regulation is critical so that people learn they can change their own arousal system. "If you get upset, take 60 breaths, focusing on the out breaths, and your brain will calm right down." Bessel van der Kolk argues that we teach kindergarten children to calm down every day by way of what some call "nap time," but once children get to the first grade, it all gets thrown out the window. By adulthood in America, the answer is to pop a pill or have a drink to calm down. Yet, the truth remains that you can achieve internal calm without alcohol or drugs.

In the science of hope, self-regulation assists with the ability to focus on goals and perform the critical thinking necessary for pathways thinking. This means self-regulation must be front and center in any strategies related to treating trauma and reducing its effects. Yoga has been successfully used in our work with adult and child survivors of trauma to help people self-regulate their bodies internal processes. We have published two studies on the beneficial effects of mindfulness and meditation practice in driving hope. This ability to self-regulate allows you to strategically focus your willpower on your valued pathways rather than depleting your mental energy on stress and anxiety.

In the summer of 2015, we started to use "hook activities" at Camp HOPE America. A hook activity is a group activity that is meant to reinforce the hope curriculum theme of the day. The activities tend to be subtler in presenting the theme and are a kinesthetic way for campers to engage with meaningful curricula. During the first week of camp each summer, programmatic details are often still being ironed out and there tend to be hiccups here and there. That first Friday, the hook activity hadn't been prepped and 20 kids were waiting in the wings. In a pinch, the Camp HOPE America Director that summer, Karianne Johansen, was asked to lead a 10-minute yoga session to fill the time. Karianne had earned her 200-hour teacher training a couple years prior and has an extensive background working with trauma-exposed youth, but she had never combined the two. Not one to back down from a challenge, she jumped in and began to lead the campers through a mindfulness and yoga session. The yoga sessions were so effective they continued every day.

Historically, Fridays are an extremely challenging day in the way of behavior at Camp HOPE America. Campers have an amazing time at camp and are then struck with the Friday reality that they are going home the following day. Like Lance at the beginning of the book, campers tend to have a rough time. It is not uncommon for multiple campers to be triggered at once on Fridays at camp. However, yoga changed things. Every camper participated in a 10-minute yoga and mindfulness exercise that involved breathing, biofeedback, and movement. That day, there was not a single behavioral issue. We saw firsthand what yoga and mindfulness could do in the minds and bodies of childhood trauma survivors. Since then, mind-body practices have become an integral part of the Camp HOPE America program, are implemented at all sites nationwide, and our success is profiled in Dr. Linda Chamberlain's website on promising practices.

Self-Empowerment Comes Second

The second crucial step according to Bessel van der Kolk is the decision that you can choose to control your own thoughts without pills or drinks. He sees programs with physical components as the most effective treatment approaches. Self-empowerment is the heart of the science of hope. The general premise is that you have the power to change things in your future by choices you make to know the sensations and feelings in your body. Engaging in movement and intentional thoughts changes the way your body feels and responds. We love Bessel's wording: "Programs with physical impact, like model mugging (a form of self-defense training), martial arts or kickboxing, or an activity that requires a range of physical effort where you actually learn to defend yourself, stand up for yourself, and feel power in your body, would be very, very effective treatments. Basically, they reinstate a sense that your organism is not a helpless tool of fate."

Expressing Your Inner Experience Comes Next

The third step is the crucial importance of telling your story, including your feelings and your inner experience. Bessel van der Kolk says, "Without being able to communicate, you're locked up inside of yourself." For many, articulating difficult emotions and experiences can prove to be extremely challenging. If the adults in your life (parents, grandparents, etc.) did not model healthy emotion identification and articulation, you may find that talk therapy is a great way to develop this skill.

Similarly, when we are able to articulate our experiences and tell our story, we can invite trustworthy people to join us in our journey. Across the board, whether it be trauma or cancer, there is more and more research and anecdotal evidence pointing toward the power of having a network of people that love and support you. In many instances, a loving and supportive community of support increases outcomes significantly.

The Final Step is Integrating Your Senses Through Rhythm

The final step may include music, dancing, drumming, or other types of sensory integration like jumping on a trampoline or moving arm in arm with a group of kids or adults. We have seen circles of children and adults do this effectively by linking arms or holding hands and singing and swaying. Many who have experienced painful traumas in life as children or adults lose their interpersonal rhythms. These types of experiences reconnect people and break through their frozen sense of separation from others. It also connects to the notion of patterned, repetitive behaviors like moving in a rocking chair that creates a soothing rhythm.

The brain-body connection is an important piece in the science of hope and mitigation of toxic stress response. Our research consistently connects mindfulness, yoga, and movement with higher hope in children and adults. In a recent publication, we reported that a six-week mindfulness/meditation training program significantly reduced stress and increased hope compared to a control group. Moreover, we have demonstrated a causal relationship showing that mindfulness practice increases hope by reducing stress.

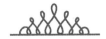

Chapter 15

Illness, Nutrition, and Hope

"Have I not commanded you? Be strong and courageous. Do not be afraid; do not be discouraged, for the Lord your God will be with you wherever you go."
—Joshua 1:9

Karianne

When I was in high school, I did a project on a missionary in Ecuador. At the time, I thought I wanted to be a missionary, so I interviewed a man named Devin about his experience. Even when I was a kid, I had a fascination with South America. Looking back on it, I can see the way that it's all woven together, but at the time it seemed like mere coincidence. I've come to believe there really are no coincidences. When I was a junior in high school, two missionaries (Margie and Baxter Swenson) from Ecuador came to our family church. Junior year was a peak year for conversations about college applications and future dreams. I had no idea where I wanted to go to school...until I met Margie and Baxter. Part of their introduction was that they ran a one-year discipleship program in Ecuador called Covenant Bible College. Immediately, a lightbulb went on for me and I knew, without a doubt, this was the path I was meant to take. I didn't even apply anywhere else! Thankfully, I was accepted and headed to Ecuador on August 25th, 2006 after I graduated from high school. Little did I know that one year in Ecuador would change the course of my entire life. I would make some of my very dearest friends and the seeds would be planted for some of the biggest challenges of my life.

My year in Ecuador was formative in countless ways. There were only 40 of us. We lived in a dorm together, had all of our classes together, and participated in regular service opportunities in a nearby rural village outside of Quito. When school wasn't in session, we traveled all over the country. Even though I was fighting homesickness, I also reveled in the glory of getting to hike through the Amazon and adventures to faraway jungle towns. A few girlfriends and I went on a trip to a town called Mindo and rode a gondola across a jungle valley and hiked for hours through the Amazon…without a guide! We were living large! Mind you, we had no cell phones when we were traveling and no Internet on campus! Life was so different in Ecuador than anywhere else I'd ever been. My faith grew as we built close relationships with each other and with local Ecuadorians that had next to nothing, yet were still faithful and trusting of a God who provides.

In addition to making some of the best friends of my life, I also made a not-so-great friend. About a month into my 8-month time in Ecuador, I got hit with a gnarly stomach bug. What I didn't realize was that it actually was *a bug—many bugs, actually. Every two weeks to the day, I was violently ill with severe gastrointestinal issues. It was glaringly obvious that my body was trying to work something out. Unbeknownst to me, that was the beginning of a ten-year health journey.*

When I got home from Ecuador, I was still getting really sick. Things mellowed a little bit, but never went away completely. I was tested for parasites and amoebas. The tests came back negative and I was given the blanket diagnosis of irritable bowel syndrome (IBS). In the naturopathic world, they refer to IBS as "intestinal bull s#%*." In the natural health realm, IBS is thought of as an M.D.'s way of saying, "Something's going on, but don't know what it is and I am not going to take the time and energy to find out." Over the course of the next few years, I did everything I could imagine to try and find relief. I eliminated gluten cold turkey. One day I woke up and literally said, "Starting today, I'm gluten-free!" A lot of my abdominal pain disappeared within days. I kept researching different diets like Paleo and GAPS (gut and psychology syndrome) and SCD (specific carbohydrate diet) and more. As time went by, my health issues continued to get worse, despite my best efforts. Issues in the GI tract don't just stay in the GI tract. They seep into other areas of our life. Within a couple years, I was wrestling with depression, anxiety, and chronic pain. I was so discouraged, frustrated, and devastated that this was my "new normal." I didn't want to accept that, so I kept looking for solutions from diets and supplements. At the end of the day, though, I had to accept the reality that life (at least at the time) wasn't the way I had pictured it.

After Ecuador, I attended Seattle Pacific University where I studied communication and music. After graduating, I had all kinds of jobs. I mentored young college women, worked at Canlis, a five-star restaurant in Seattle, worked at Mount Hermon, a summer camp in the Santa Cruz Mountains, became a yoga instructor, started a jewelry business, and later spent summers working at Camp HOPE America with trauma-exposed children. Many of my friends were working their dream jobs and I envied them. I still hadn't felt like I had found "my thing." I remember having a conversation with a friend when I was about 24. "I feel like God has a huge calling for me—like I am capable of greatness and it's right around the corner…but I don't know what it is yet." As my health journey continued, I wondered if I would go down the holistic health road. I even looked at Bastyr University's naturopathic doctor program in Kenmore, Washington. But the lie kept rolling around in my head, "I'm not smart enough to do something like that." I hoped my self-talk wasn't true, but it sure felt like it was.

Even though I was battling some difficult physical and mental health issues, people regularly commented on my joy and sparkle. There were definitely days when I felt good and "sparkly," but there was also an undercurrent of depression. To this day, I find it amazing that we have the emotional capacity to both experience grief and joy in the same moment.

Since I was a child, I have been deeply empathetic. When I was a kid, I couldn't put words to it. Empathy manifested itself as an emotional roller coaster and a sea of emotion when I was a kid. A lot of times, my parents didn't quite know how to handle me because I was feeling all manner of things so deeply. I felt the emotions of other people and often took them on as if they were my own. There were times in life that I felt like I was carrying the weight of the world. I'd sense the depression of a friend, the suicidal thoughts of a stranger, the marital problems of adults, and the shame that often accompanies sexual abuse…it felt like I had lived a thousand lives. It was a blessing and a gift, but it felt like a curse a lot of the time. In my 20s, though, I started to realize that my empathy made me powerful in my work with adults and children impacted by trauma. Through lots of work with various therapists, I learned how to differentiate between my own emotions and the emotions of others. That work had been born out of desperation because my body was holding all of this emotional trauma, whether it was mine or someone else's. All the while, the intestinal chaos continued and I grew apathetic and resentful that I hadn't experienced healing. I started to believe that I never would be healthy again.

After years of being fiercely independent and loving the single life, I met Mike. He quickly earned the nickname of "Sweet Mike" because of his sensitivity, deep thinking, thoughtfulness, and artistic side. He, too, worked with at-risk youth and our gifts and passions aligned in a really perfect and beautiful way. When we met, I was sure that Mike was "too nice" for me. It turns out that A) I deserve to be treated well (that was new to me in relationships) and B) I was going to need a strong, sensitive, gentle, compassionate man by my side in the years to come. We got engaged in November of 2015. I bawled my eyes out the day after we got engaged. My intestinal issues were at an all-time high and my mental health was suffering in a huge way. It turns out that gut health is directly related to mental health because of how many of our neurotransmitters are made in the GI tract. Gut health quickly gives way to anxiety and depression because we don't have the neurotransmitters that we need to be happy and stable. On a December night in 2015, Mike took me to the ER for serious GI issues. Bless his heart—he heard me talk about some really graphic things and yet still looked at me with adoration and compassion. I needed him. "In sickness and in health" started long before we said "I do." We picked our wedding colors in the ER that night.

Shortly thereafter, I was finally diagnosed with giardia. I was overjoyed! Parasite panels can often give a false negative, which explains why my initial test eight years earlier had showed that I was "fine." I immediately named the parasite so that I could talk to it and tell it that we were breaking up. You've gotta keep your sense of humor with these kinds of things! A heavy dose of antibiotics followed and I soon tested "negative" for giardia—Brutus Rex Shiitake was dead! Good news, right? Even though Brutus was dead, I still felt terrible. My intestines were extremely damaged from a long-term infection. The world kept spinning and in November 2015, I started working full-time as the Camp HOPE America Director, a job that I was passionate about and felt confident in though I still felt there was some other calling in my future.

Mike and I got married in March of 2016. We worked at camp together over the summer. My health kept declining. I pushed through, but I was not doing well. In October, 2017, I woke up one day to find a lump on my neck. Mike and I had barely been married six months. Tests were ordered, many of them inconclusive. It was decided to do a needle biopsy on my neck to rule out lymphoma. I went to the biopsy alone, thinking that it would be a quick, casual procedure. When the physician showed me the CT scan that revealed the mass in my neck, I had a profound spiritual experience. I should have been terrified that I might have cancer, but I found peace instead. The lump on my neck was the shape of a heart. A wave washed over my body and I felt, "You're not alone. I am with you. There will be purpose in this. I promise." A week later, I got a call from my doctor. "Most of the cells that were extracted are necrotic, so they can't be tested." "What does that mean?" I asked. "It means that the cells were dead. We need to schedule you for surgery right away to get a bigger chunk of the mass so that we can actually test it."

There was nothing hopeful or positive in the ominous finding, but I felt strangely calm. A couple weeks later, I had surgery to remove the enlarged lymph nodes to test them further. The mass was wrapped around my carotid artery and was entangled in nerves, so removing it had the potential for life-threatening consequences and permanent nerve damage. But they got enough to test. Days of anticipation and anxiety followed as we waited to get the pathology results.

On December 2, 2016, I was told that I had lymphoma. The oncological surgeon and Pathology team, however, were all stumped as to what kind of lymphoma I had. So, they sent my results to Stanford University in an attempt to unveil the mystery of the biopsy. Two more weeks passed. The Stanford results came back. I had a "rare and aggressive" form of lymphoma called Grey Zone Lymphoma (GZL). GZL affects less than 300 people in the United States. I've always been pretty unique, so it was strangely unsurprising that I would have a unique and uncommon form of cancer. Internet research brought no comfort because there are so few cases that there are not any clinical trials to look at regarding treatment or outcomes. The case reports are not good.

I'd read so much on the Internet about what people wish they would've known before starting chemo, how to cope with hair loss, etc. People talked about naming their cancer, so I named mine "Lawrence" and named my chemo pump "Xena" (like Xena Warrior Princess!). I was faced with the question of how I would respond to this. Would I respond in anger? In action? In fear? In anxiety? In power? With hope? I trusted God when he told me He would use it and that He would be with me. I rested in that belief every single day. I trusted that He could and would heal me and this was the way He was going to do it. No matter what, though, I knew that God was a healer—when and how He decided to heal me wasn't my decision to make.

Major Illness and Hope

Major illness can have a significant and negative impact on hope. Initially, we might all assume that major illness would only negatively impact hope because it is frustrating at its best and devastating at its worst. Devastation *must* destroy hope, right? Not exactly. Remember, you can have a high Hope score if you have a goal, a pathway, and agency. Therefore, if a person receives a devastating diagnosis, but there is a viable and promising treatment option, that devastating diagnosis doesn't necessarily destroy hope. It may actually increase hope! When we talk about major illness and hope, we are talking more about the physiological effects of major illness on hope—both negative and positive.

We asked Karianne to help us think in this chapter about the trauma of major illness, related issues around nutrition, and the neurobiology of hope. Her insights can help anyone processing either specific trauma or a major illness and provide a deeper understanding of how the body deals with it and what we can do to feed the body in a healthy way during the process.

Our bodies' innate intelligence often has answers that we don't have. Our body may be aware of an infection that we never become aware of. The same innate intelligence often allows our bodies to fight battles that we are completely unaware of like Karianne's giardia. However, these battles are not fought without sacrifice. One of the amazing systems of our bodies is our Autonomic Nervous System (ANS). Within the ANS, there are two subdivisions: the sympathetic division and the parasympathetic division. The sympathetic state is activated in times of stress. One way to remember this is to think of how *sympathy* is often expressed toward a person that is in a time or season of stress. For example, our Paleolithic ancestors were catapulted into a sympathetic state when they were being chased by a saber-toothed tiger or physically fighting their enemies. Our bodies are designed to utilize the sympathetic state when it is needed for survival. In this state, the body's primary concern is *short-term* survival. This is the state in which the "fight, flight, or freeze" response takes place that we touched on earlier. Imagine this. If you are running for your life from a large animal, how important would digestion be? How important would it be to make sex hormones? How important would your immune system be? The answer…not very important. If you are running from a tiger, what you need is to run fast, to have superhuman strength and energy, and to be able to access adequate amounts of oxygen while running for your life.

In the sympathetic state, your heart rate increases, blood flow moves away from non-essential systems like digestion and moves to large muscles groups, like the leg and arm muscles, necessary for "running from the tiger." The bronchial tubes, that we inhale air through, dilate so that more air and oxygen can be consumed at rapid speeds. Even urinary output decreases. Digestion halts along with the production of sex hormones. Digestion and sex hormones are completely unimportant when you are running for your life. And how inconvenient would it be to need to use the restroom in a moment like that? Even though you've likely never run from a deadly animal, it is likely that you have experienced this effect. Have you ever been nervous for a big presentation? You likely found that the "nervous tummy" that preceded your presentation went away entirely for the duration of the presentation itself. Your heart was probably pounding. Your blood pressure probably went up. Then, you got in "the zone." You completely forgot that your neck had been tense all day. Physiologically, your body may as well have been running from a saber-toothed tiger. The same physiological responses were taking place, but they had a completely different cause.

Just like a saber-toothed tiger can trigger the sympathetic state, so can our everyday physical stress. That physical stress may be the presence of environmental toxins, an underlying dental infection, gastrointestinal inflammation, undetected food allergies, undiagnosed cancer, or autoimmune conditions, along with a host of other issues. Have you ever had a season of life where you felt as though you couldn't calm down? Where relaxation was next to impossible? Chances are that you either had mental and emotional stress in abundance *or* your body was dealing with a major "body burden." In our harried society, "body burdens" are becoming more and more common as our environments are increasingly more toxic. Physiological stresses such as major illnesses cause the activation of the sympathetic nervous system and all of the implications that come along with it. There are two important implications. Digestion and nutrient absorption worsens and the body becomes hypervigilant and struggles to fall asleep and rest. Our bodies think they are running from a tiger, so sleep can wait!

The parasympathetic state, on the other hand, has completely different functions and processes. In a parasympathetic state, the heart rate slows down, bronchial tubes constrict to their normal size, blood pressure normalizes, saliva production increases, the stomach produces more hydrochloric acid for digestion, and muscles relax. In the visioning exercise, we just did in the last chapter, if you did it well, you were primarily operating in your parasympathetic state. You were calm and relaxed and there was no saber-tooth tiger—real or imagined.

If you have participated in conversations about digestion or nutrient absorption, you may have heard the phrase "rest and digest." Digestion is a process of the parasympathetic state. In short, if our bodies are chronically stressed, we will not produce the acids and enzymes that our bodies need to appropriately break down food and make it absorbable. We have the ability to activate our parasympathetic nervous system. Deep belly breathing is a favorite for many people that are aiming at relaxation. For some, something like getting a massage will turn on their parasympathetic nervous system. For others, it's going for a walk. Writing can be an effective tool as well. There are many ways to bring about this state. Our job is to learn how to do it so that we can allow our bodies the time to heal, rest, digest, and relax. To fully understand why we need to take charge of our responses to stress, we need to talk about nutrition and its role in mental health whether during a major illness or in everyday living.

Nutrition and Hope

Nutrition plays a powerful role in whether we are experiencing rising or falling hope. The adage "you are what you eat" is more than a phrase used to shame people for eating dessert. Quite literally, we become what we eat. While your rear end won't turn into the cinnamon rolls you ate for breakfast, those cinnamon rolls will be used as fuel by nearly every cell in your body. Similarly, a meal full of nutrients will be used for fuel by nearly every cell in your body. And while it is true that we are what we eat, what is even more true is that we are what we absorb.

The absorption of nutrients is a beautiful and complicated process that could be talked about for many chapters. However, for the purposes of this book, we will talk about it from a foundational level. Essentially, the process of digestion is a process of the parasympathetic nervous system. During a relaxed parasympathetic state, the sight, smell, and even the *thought* of food can bring about saliva production (a necessary component of healthy digestion), the secretion of hydrochloric acid (HCl) by the stomach, and the digestive domino effect that includes digestive enzymes along with multiple hormones that are vital in the process of breaking down food to be used by the body for energy. Without the digestive system working properly (starting with the brain and then trickling down), we are in danger of being fed, but not nourished. One equivalent would be putting gas in your car, but having a hole in your gas tank. If you don't heal the hole in your gas tank, no matter how much gas you put in your car, you are going to be running on empty.

As we discussed earlier, digestion takes a break during a stressed or sympathetic state. The body's ability to produce vital digestive components becomes impaired because those components are considered "non-essential" compared to what our bodies interpret as "survival mode." In our fast-paced society, our sympathetic state is triggered by events that are far from life-threatening—traffic on the way to work, an argument with a spouse, a work deadline, our children acting out, a broken relationship, etc. But, our bodies are also triggered into this state from trauma, which can often be life-threatening. Trauma of all kinds impacts the nervous system, which impacts the digestive system, which impacts nutrient absorption, which impacts the production of neurotransmitters, which impacts cellular health as well as mental health. Our mental health plays a large role in how hopeful or apathetic we are. Just like chronic fear and hope can't coexist indefinitely, neither can chronic depression and hope. When we take a step back and understand how the systems of our bodies work, we see that they are intricately woven together.

Our bodies are made up of tiny cells that rely on neurotransmitters to function properly. Neurotransmitters are, essentially, messengers. Their job is to help nerve cells communicate with each other. As such, they are vital to our overall health as well as our mental health. These messengers don't come out of nowhere, though. Neurotransmitters are, for the most part, made from amino acids. Amino acids are the result of the digestive breakdown of protein by the body. Similarly, our bodies' muscle proteins use amino acids as their building blocks.

When we don't properly digest and absorb our food, we miss out on many of the nutrients that would otherwise be readily accessible and utilized. Fatty acids are the building blocks of hormones that catalyze all kinds of processes in the body. Without proper absorption, we can't make those hormones and the rest of the chain reaction gets altered negatively. When it comes to amino acids, there are two types—essential and non-essential. Nonessential amino acids can be created by the body whereas essential amino acids cannot be made by the body and must be obtained through food. So, why does it matter if we are missing out on amino acids? Well, in addition to being the building blocks for muscle protein, amino acids are the precursors to the majority of neurotransmitters. Some examples of neurotransmitters include serotonin, which we know to be largely responsible for mood, sleep, memory, sexual desire/function, and more. The amino acid tryptophan is a precursor to serotonin. Similarly, other amino acids are required to produce neurotransmitters like adrenaline, noradrenaline, dopamine, and many others. Dopamine is commonly known to relate to the "pleasure center" of the brain. Dopamine is responsible for a "runner's high." What else would enable a person to feel elated after many miles of hitting the pavement?

In their book *Why Stomach Acid is Good for You*, Drs. Jonathan Wright and Lane Lenard discuss the role of neurotransmitters in depression. In Dr. Wright's clinical practice, he has found that amino acid supplementation is as effective, if not more effective, than treating depression with patented antidepressants. While supplementing with an amino acid complex can be extremely helpful, it does not solve the likely issues—poor nutrient absorption. Dr. Wright is a huge proponent of aiming to fix the digestive process as a means of dealing with the root cause of many issues including depression. Imagine if your diet doesn't even have those essential amino acids present in the first place—you are at an extreme disadvantage in overcoming depression or low energy and low hope issues in your life.

At Camp HOPE America, we have seen drastic differences in our campers depending on what we feed them. At most locations, the meals consist of typical "camp food," which kids love, but that makes health-conscious adults cringe—tater tots, macaroni and cheese, corndogs, French fries…basically, meals with little to no nutritional value. Conversely, there are a very small handful of locations that serve real food—salad, BBQ chicken, avocado, vegetables, and sometimes even steak! As you might guess, the behavior that we see from children that are being fed real food is in stark contrast to the tater tot-fueled campers.

The campers that are eating real food trigger less, are better behaved, and there is little inter-cabin conflict. That description only scratches the surface of the observable differences. Real food positively impacts their mental health because it contains essential amino acids that are necessary to produce important neurotransmitters along with a multitude of vitamins and minerals that are missing from standard "camp food." By feeding campers real food, we are giving campers the very best chance at absorbing nutrients that will properly fuel their bodies and their brains. Diets that are high in refined carbohydrates, sugars, and processed foods are a highly unlikely source of amino acids. So, if poor digestion and nutrient absorption impairs the body's ability to assimilate amino acids, which are later converted into neurotransmitters, where does that leave us? That often leaves us with deficiencies that cause chronic depression and anxiety to creep in and slowly rob us of hope.

Is Processed Sugar a Pathway to Hope?

A few hope researchers over the years have talked about having a candy bowl in your office at work to increase hope in employees. Others have done experiments to see how small sugary rewards tends to increase motivation in children or adults. This is stupid. Processed sugar is not a pathway to hope. In fact, the opposite is true. Sugar is a short-term high coupled with a long-term low. Sugar like anything else in moderation is not bad for you. Glucose is an important energy source for the brain—our hope engine. Glucose is a simple sugar that your body welcomes without major problems. It stimulates the pancreas to produce insulin and this helps your brain realize that you are now less hungry than before you ate. Too much glucose can cause problems including the challenge your liver has in processing it, but, at least with glucose, our body has a mechanism to tell us when to stop.

The real sugar problem is high fructose corn syrup (HFCS). Our diets are saturated with HFCS. If you don't believe it, the next time you go to the grocery store or Costco check out the ingredients on EVERY type of processed food and see just how many have HFCS. It will be demoralizing, then you will get mad, then you will come back and read this part of the book again!

Fructose is not a friend of your Hope score. Fructose does not stimulate the pancreas and therefore it never tells your brain that you have had enough. You can eat an entire bag of Halloween candy and never receive any 'cease and desist' messages from your brain. Fructose can only be metabolized by the liver. This means that three times as many calories are running through the liver with fructose than with glucose. If you have high cholesterol, the primary culprit is usually too much fructose. If you have hypertension or high blood pressure, you guessed it, probably too much uric acid which is produced from too much fructose running through your liver.

Nutrition matters in the context of hope. People with low hope might gravitate toward caffeine or sugar to temporarily give them higher levels of energy and motivation to pursue goals each day. It is a bad idea. Fructose changes the way your brain understands your consumption levels. Short explanation: Your brain does not know you are full and your metabolism is overwhelmed as you eat more and more. We recently swore off sugary sodas in our quest for hope. Why? Soda contains high rates of fructose and you can consume a lot of it without ever feeling full. Then, one day you wake fat, hungry, and excited for more sugar!

Major illness and nutrition issues can all impact our ability to live daily with high hope. The bottom-line: More exercise, more fruits, vegetables, and meat, and less fructose is the best pathway to rising hope.

What happens when your own nutrition and health issues begin to destroy you from within? Whether it is cancer, or stress, or other health issues, you can choose to look for the opportunity to make different choices around nutrition. You should think more about the food you feed your body and the ways you can see your illness as an opportunity for hope.

Low hope can come from physical illness or chronic pain in our lives. Karianne said her low hope through ten years of health issues came as she lost the ability to find a pathway out of the pain and illness. After ten years of health struggles in her life, she was despairing of ever finding a pathway to health. She had tried everything over the years.

When word came of her cancer diagnosis, Karianne's family was devastated. Karianne said she was "relieved." She said, "I feel like I was given a bow and arrow a long time ago when I started getting sick. When I was given that bow and arrow, though, I was also blindfolded. I've spent years pulling back the bow and shooting arrows with no idea of where the target is or if there even *is* a target at all. The blindfold has now been removed and I'm strong now from years of pulling back the bow and shooting arrows. Now I knew exactly where the target was and I was ready to shoot with all my strength from years of blind practice." There was finally something to fight. There was an explanation for her pain. She had something she could set a goal around and begin looking for a pathway through. Karianne had been sick for so long that a devastating cancer diagnosis was a relief.

Here is the rest of her story.

Karianne's Journey Through Grey Zone Lymphoma

On December 15, 2016, I had an appointment with Dr. Marin Xavier, one of the leading lymphoma specialists on the West Coast at Scripps Mercy Hospital. "I live to treat these kinds of cancers," Dr. Xavier said, as she took my hand. She became my oncologist when Mike and I moved down to San Diego. "You shouldn't wait any more than three weeks to start chemotherapy." I listened intently as Dr. Xavier described the chemotherapy regimen that she would recommend along with all of its short- and long-term side effects. It would total 576 hours of dose-adjusted E-POCH, meaning each 96-hour infusion would be inpatient at the hospital and would be increased by 20% each time. Dose-adjusted E-POCH is just about as aggressive as chemotherapy can be. The nurses fear even a drop on their body, because it will burn a hole in their skin. When you've got a big, scary cancer, you pull out the big guns to treat it. Even with this chemo regimen, Dr. Xavier could only guarantee a 60% survival rate. That's barely better than half! That wasn't good enough for me. I dove head first into researching any and every single thing that I could do to weaken my cancer cells and make them more susceptible to the oxidative damage of chemotherapy.

There is a proliferation index called Ki-67 that pathology labs run on cancer cells to measure how fast they are growing. The scale is 0 to 100. When oncologists see a Ki-67 in the 80s, they are almost always met with a PET Scan that shows metastasized cancer all throughout the body that has caused multiple organ failures and massive illness. My Ki-67 was 90. A 90 on this index shows that the cancer has been growing and gaining momentum for a long time. The first oncologist I saw had never even seen a 90 on this index. He had also never heard of Grey Zone Lymphoma—that's how rare it is. "Your PET Scan and your pathology results don't match. You should have cancer all over your body…but you don't. All of it is above your diaphragm, which indicates that you're Stage 2." After discussing my health history with this oncologist, it became apparent that my parasitic "friend" Brutus had activated my immune system so much that it was fighting hard against the cancer for a very long time. Once the giardia was gone, the aggressive cancer bulldozed my immune system and manifested externally almost overnight in the form of a mass.

Mike and I were living in the San Francisco Bay Area when I was diagnosed. We couldn't afford our apartment if I wasn't able to work. We started packing our first apartment together on Christmas night and moved to San Diego to live with my parents and I started chemo within a week and a half. It was time to battle.

On January 9, 2017, I started chemotherapy. The start of the journey was quite tumultuous given the chaos and disorganization of the medical system. But, I kept my spirits up as much as I could. In the hospital, there's a definite vibe of "Be nice to the nurses and the nurses will be nice to you." Since each round was five days, I figured I'd better make some friends! After about 7 hours of waiting, the first chemotherapy bags were hung. Five days in the hospital flew by with lots of visits from family and friends. I was thrilled to be discharged from the hospital after five days without fresh air or sunshine. Within 30 minutes of leaving the hospital, the side effects started setting in. My throat swelled, my head pounded, my body began to feel like one giant bruise, and I could barely stand long enough to take my first shower in a week. The two weeks of recovery at home were riddled with all kinds of pain and chemo-related issues.

The Internet is a very powerful thing and can do different things for different people. For me, it was a place of empowerment and action. A couple days before round 2, I watched a documentary about cancer. The documentary provided some scary information about the short- and long-term side effects of cancer and the way that allopathic medicine can downplay these often-permanent side effects. This was arguably the only time that I truly freaked out during my cancer journey. I immediately scheduled a Skype appointment with a well-known naturopathic doctor. "How do I protect myself from the toxicity of chemo? What can I do?" I had never heard of her recommendation— therapeutic fasting and a Ketogenic diet. Round 2 started the following day, so there was no time to waste. I started eating as much fat as I could get my hands on in order to comply with a high fat, low carb Ketogenic diet.

Before I started chemo, I put together a Pinterest board that I named "Crafting through Chemo." I had all kinds of tutorials on things like cross-stitching, embroidery, and all kinds of other crafts that could be done from bed. If I was going to feel like crap, I was at least going to make some cute stuff in the meantime. I had gone to Michael's craft store in preparation. To this day, the crafting supplies sit in a bag, untouched. Crafts could wait. My life was on the line. I spent every free moment that I had researching and studying and learning. I got to use myself as a guinea pig. I'm confident that the changes that I implemented and the disciplines that I put into practice played a significant role in saving my life and maximizing chemo's impact while minimizing the detrimental effects.

One of the practices that I implemented was therapeutic fasting. For rounds 3, 4, 5, and 6 of chemo, I fasted for at least 48 hours beforehand. USC had recently come out with research about the protective mechanisms of fasting and the way that it weakens cancer cells and protects healthy cells. Their results were astounding. Sign me up! I also utilized natural detox therapies and discovered the power of essential oils for pain management. I could literally feel my primary mass shrinking after each round of chemotherapy. This was obviously something to celebrate, especially given that a lot of GZL patients will have disease progression even while undergoing chemotherapy. Two *rounds of chemo brought about a 50% decrease of cancer activity. After four rounds, I had another PET Scan to monitor progress. The day that I started round 5, Dr. Xavier cheerfully exclaimed, "Good news all around!" My mom had come with me to the appointment. We looked at each other with slight confusion. "Your scan is all clear!" We immediately burst into tears of joy. I was declared cancer-free on April 5th, 2017. Dr. Xavier was very pleased with the scan, of course, but explained that I would still need to do two more rounds of chemotherapy as "insurance."*

After a total of 576 hours of chemotherapy, I was discharged from the hospital for the last time on April 29th. My entire extended family plus dozens of family friends surprised me at the hospital. In classic Karianne fashion, I danced out of the hospital in a purple, sparkly leotard with the Destiny Child's song "I'm a Survivor" playing full blast. Scripps Mercy Hospital had never seen such a triumphant and joyful exit. We took the place by storm. It was rare for the oncology nurses to celebrate remission with patients at all. By the time that cancer patients were doing in-patient chemo like I was doing, it was either a last-ditch effort or it was palliative care. It was nearly unheard of to see oncology patients walk out of the hospital cancer-free. And yet, it happened. I worked my tail off—changing my diet, managing stress, implementing a crazy amount of self-care practices, while continuing to trust God. My self-talk changed too. It was official. I was a survivor. I had been a survivor for nearly ten years, but I was finally a cancer-free survivor.

The journey to fully restored health is a long one that Karianne is still on and will continue to be on for several years to come. But her body is slowly healing and her constitution is more powerful and her spirit is more hopeful than it has ever been.

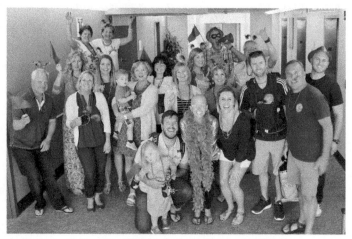

Karianne finishing chemotherapy (2017)

Karianne chose hope even in the face of her fears. She could have lived in the dark shadow of anxiety. She could have obsessed over the bad cards she was dealt. But she made a conscious, courageous choice to set goals whenever she had any control, to identify and re-evaluate pathways repeatedly as her goals needed to change, and to lean on her friends and family members even when her hope waned.

Today, Karianne is turning her pain into power. She has become a Certified Nutritional Therapy Practitioner and is working with fellow cancer fighters and survivors to equip and empower them for their battles—using her own courage to help others find courage to help others find courage, using her own high hope to help others face their fears and choose hope. Because of the pain and adversity in her own life, she has found her calling. You can contact her and learn more about her work with cancer patients at: www.inspirawellnesscollective.com.

But what if the enemy is just the day to day stressors of life? What if the enemy is the broken dishwasher or the car that won't start? What if the attacker of your soul tomorrow is someone in your parking spot at work or the road rage guy in front of you on the way home from work?

Karianne's use of a Ketogenic diet during chemo inspired us and many others to learn more about it. As Casey faced health issues about six months after Karianne finished chemo, his San Diego cardiologist, Dr. Bret Scher, challenged Casey to try a Ketogenic diet. Casey hired Karianne to help him navigate a pathway to weight loss, lower cholesterol, lower blood pressure, and elimination of all pharmaceutical products from his daily diet! As you evaluate your own life in the context of health and wellness, don't be afraid to look at the Ketogenic diet and other options. If you decide to make changes, hire a good nutritionist and consult with your doctor, but you can make changes that will build your immune system up after trauma, illness, or other adversity!

Karianne and her husband Mike navigated her cancer successfully by setting goals and finding pathways – with the support of many caring and loving family members and friends. But the best part of the story is still being written. They are now parents to a beautiful baby boy. On June 13, 2019, after surviving chemo and cancer, Karianne gave birth to a 12 pound, 10 ounce boy named Bennett.

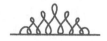

Chapter 16

Is AT&T an Enemy of Hope?

"Do you want to play a game?"
—**The Machine** in movie *War Games* (1983)

War Games

The 1983 movie War Games is a fictional account of the United States Air Force Strategic Missile Wing controllers at NORAD deciding to automate the missile launch controls for nuclear war. Control is given to a NORAD supercomputer with the goal of running simulations until it eliminates the chance for nuclear war. The simulator is called the War Operation Plan Response (WOPR).

    David, a high hope high school computer hacker from Seattle, is using his computer to hack into his school's computer system to change his poor grades and then does the same for a friend. Then, they decide to hack into a computer gaming company. During his misguided effort, he gets into a game called "Global Thermonuclear War." It seems interesting enough but he struggles to get access to the game. Once he learns about "backdoors" and sees that one of the games is called "Falken's Maze," he decides to guess on the backdoor password. Soon, he realizes that Stephen Falken, an early artificial intelligence researcher had a son named Joshua. David guesses "Joshua" is the password for his "Global Thermonuclear War" game.

David doesn't realize it is not a game. He has hacked into NORAD and starts playing his game as the "Soviet Union." The NORAD computer plays with David and convinces NORAD that the Soviets are really releasing submarines and bombers and getting ready to start World War III. The DEFCON level rises as the world appears to move toward nuclear war. The threat is not real but the stress levels from the perceived threat are like someone running from a bear in the woods when there is no bear.

David, the teenager, ends up getting arrested and faces espionage charges. He is brought to NORAD but then escapes, travels to Oregon, and now, obsessed with Stephen Falken, finds him convinced that nuclear war really is inevitable. WOPR is going to start World War III and David must figure out how to beat the computer simulator with the help of its creator Stephen Falken. The WOPR computer stages a massive Soviet first strike within the simulator that is so real that NORAD is preparing an actual retaliatory strike against the Soviets. But WOPR overrides NORAD systems and tries to launch the missiles. Now, the machine is playing with itself. Humans have lost control. Eventually, the machine discovers the concept of mutual assured destruction and finds nuclear war is a "strange game" and the "only winning move is not to play." The DEFCON level returns to normal and the world survives.

The day to day stressors of life sometimes become bigger than life. We can lose our perspective and frustration can drive us to unhealthy places mentally and emotionally. When this happens, hope goes low and it is hard to get it back quickly.

The Defense Readiness Condition (DEFCON) is the alert state used by the United States Armed Forces. It was developed by the Joint Chiefs of Staff. It prescribes five graduated levels of readiness or states of alert for the U.S. military. DEFCON 5 is for normal peacetime status. DEFCON 1 takes us to global severity, like nuclear war. As human beings longing for hope in our lives, we too can sometimes find ourselves on a similar DEFCON scale when things don't go well even amidst the everyday frustrations of life.

A few months ago, Casey went to DEFCON1 trying to solve a home Internet-service problem with AT&T. Days later, his family would joke about his frustration and "maniacal laughter" after three hours of being passed around inside AT&T over a two-day period. For the first few days though after it happened, it was…too soon. Could AT&T be an enemy of hope? Probably not, but his journey is a great example of how obstacles to agency, goals, and pathways in a real-life situation can impact hope and create enormous frustration and anger. Remember that anger/frustration is a natural, normal result/response when our expectations don't match our lived experience in life situations.

One day last fall, the Gwinn family lost their home Internet due an undiagnosed problem. Motivation to get it fixed was high. Over a period of days, each family member called to try to get the problem fixed. Casey's wife, Beth called. She really needed to connect to work from home. Casey's daughter Karianne called. She needed it for her online classes for her Nutritional Therapy program. His son-in-law Mike called. He needed to work on his graduate school application. Each time, they would talk to a different person. Repair appointments were scheduled. Days went by. The Internet still did not work. Finally, after two weeks without Internet, AT&T identified the problem—it was the cables under the street in front of the house. AT&T had not installed an access point, so the cables were completely inaccessible. A contractor would need to be hired, permits would need to be issued. Time estimate: Maybe a few days but nothing was firm. Gwinn Goal: Get the Internet working; Agency (Motivation): Very high; Pathways: Not necessarily under the Gwinn family's control.

At dinner that night, the whole family asked Casey to intervene with AT&T because they had all failed. Casey saw their frustration and thought: "How can this be that hard to solve?" He entered the family challenge with high hope. The goal? Find some way to get Internet—By expediting the repair schedule? With a Hot Spot? By increasing capacity on his daughter's AT&T personal cell phone? Upgrading to DSL service instead of AT&T U-Verse? There were many options/solutions to the problem. Casey began his first call with "Vishnu" in "Technical Support" for AT&T at 9 PM. *An hour later*, Vishnu announced that there was "No estimate" for a repair time on the U-Verse Internet. He recommended Casey call in the morning to talk to the "Retention Team" and gave him a "direct" number to call. Frustration grew because one pathway was blocked, but others were still available. Gwinn Goal: Get some type of Internet; Agency (Motivation): Still high; Pathways: Unclear but with options to think through and possibly pursue. DEFCON4.

The next morning, Casey, with a high level of determination, placed his call to the "Retentions Team." "Jaunice" took Casey's call and he explained the problem and the need for a solution. AT&T was still billing the Gwinn family for Internet even though they had none. AT&T needed to stop billing for it and/or provide another option. After nearly 45 minutes on the phone, Jaunice told Casey that AT&T could install DSL—a faster Internet option than U-Verse but since she was not in that department, she offered to transfer him directly. Minutes later, however, Casey was again entering his phone number and giving a password to a "Customer Service" representative. Her name was "Love" but Casey was not feeling any. "Love" explained that she was not in "DSL Technical Support" and therefore could not help him. After 20 minutes, she offered to transfer him to DSL directly. She said her "best friend" worked in DSL and she would transfer him directly to her. After the transfer, Casey was again back at the beginning, entering his phone number and password. Casey never met Love's "best friend." Eventually, he ended up with a new representative named "Raymond." After 30 minutes on the phone, Raymond told Casey that DSL was probably not a solution but he would transfer him to "DSL Sales", not DSL Technical Support to confirm whether DSL was possible. DEFCON3.

After again ending up going through phone number and password entry, "Paul" from DSL Sales was on the phone talking from a loud boiler room that sound like home to hundreds of operators and explained to Casey that he could not hear him and told him to talk louder. Soon, Casey's voice was rising and Paul kept saying "You need to talk louder." After 15 minutes, Paul said that the Gwinns could not get DSL because they did not choose it when they signed up for AT&T and therefore they were disqualified from having it at all. Paul told Casey he would transfer him directly to "Wireless" to get a hot spot added to his daughter's phone. Do you know what is coming now? Phone number and password entered. A sweet woman announces "Wireless"—no name provided. Within minutes, she ruled out adding capacity to Karianne's phone to provide Internet access and said that a separate "hot spot" would require a two-year contract. She said there was nothing in the AT&T online records to say that AT&T should have to provide such a "hot spot" for free or limited cost or duration. She said she was transferring Casey to "Customer Loyalty" and that they would solve the problem for him. The nameless Wireless representative, of course, offered a direct transfer so Casey did not have to start over by entering his phone number and password. Five minutes later, Casey was entering his phone number and password again and waiting for a representative. DEFCON2.

"Chris" came on the phone after a 3-minute delay and introduced himself as a "Customer Loyalty" representative. He knew nothing of the Gwinn Family situation. Casey had to tell the story from the beginning all over again. Chris listened to the story for about two minutes and then interrupted Casey. "I am ready to cancel your Internet service pursuant to your request." "I don't want to cancel our service. I want (goal) AT&T to give us another solution to getting Internet Service in our home since we don't know when you can repair the problem in the street outside our house but you are still charging us!" "There is no need to get frustrated, Mr. Gwinn. I will cancel your Internet service pursuant to your request." Blood pressure, not hope rising. "What does it mean that you are in 'Customer Loyalty' if your only option is to cancel our service?" "Mr. Gwinn, I am here to solve your problem. What day would like your Internet service to stop?" Casey was beside himself. He hung up on Chris. DEFCON1. Fire the nukes.

Two days later, Casey received his new, monthly AT&T bill for the inoperable Gwinn Family Internet service.

Final Hope Assessment? Goal: Still clear—Get Internet; Agency (Motivation): Almost gone; Pathways: None. Falling Hope score—like a lead balloon. First, hope. Then, anger. Then, despair. Then, apathy. Remember what apathy is? At the end, Casey didn't care about anything anymore—not his wife's work, not his son-in-law's graduate school applications, not his daughter's Nutrition classes, not the Internet, and not AT&T.

We will share the end of the AT&T story later in the book. AT&T may not be the enemy, but there may be times in life when we simply cannot achieve a viable, healthy goal no matter how hard we try. Even in those moments though, we must still make the effort to nurture hope back to life.

Nurturing Hope

Imagination is an instrument of hope! The essence of hope is your ability to understand the way things are right now, and to imagine the way the future could be. One of the greatest gifts a parent can give a child is the gift of imagination—imagining that things are different or can be different. John Lennon's "Imagine" was a song about hope! If you can imagine something, you can begin to think about ways for your imagined idea to become a reality or become closer to reality. Now, let's look at how this gets applied in the nurturing of hope.

Casey and his wife told stories to their children at bedtime. Sometimes those stories were books but often they were made up stories. As the children got older, they too could join in making up the story. The use of imagination to learn to make up stories is a great foundation for a high hope child.

Stage 1 (Goal Setting): To begin nurturing hope, the desirable goal must be described in specific detail and exist within the realm of possible attainment. We suggest this first step should not be rushed. If anything, err on the side of spending too much time on goal identification. If you are working with another person, it is worth asking for clarification and detail. This will allow their imagination of the goal to flourish. This initial stage of goal clarification tends to temporarily increase the agency dimension of hope allowing for focus on pathways development. To be clear, if you want to nourish hope, you first must build agency (motivation) toward the goal.

Many times, children, when asked what they want to be, will answer "A professional basketball player" or "A professional soccer player." This may or may not be in the realm of possible attainment! A further goal setting conversation may also be helpful as you ask them what other goals they might have if they are not able to become a professional athlete. This will help them create alternatives for their future, without spending all their energy on a goal that may not be attainable. If your goal setting is about re-goaling, this may take even more time based on the frustration of failing at the original goal. Once Casey failed to get AT&T to give him another option for Internet, he needed to identify another way to get Internet (a new goal).

Stage 2 (Pathway Focus): Viable pathways to goal attainment can be developed with specific attention to measurable benchmarks. Benchmarks can serve as an important feedback system allowing us to self-regulate behavior and emotions. One way we have found useful is to start with the goal and work backward in time. For example, if your goal is to be a professor at a major university, you need to get an interview. Before you can get an interview, you need to have a strong curricula vita or resume. To have a strong vita, you need to publish and present research. And so on, working backward to the point where the future can become connected to the present. As this example demonstrates, ultimate goals always have steps (smaller goals) in the journey.

While working on this stage personally or with others, we should be encouraged to consider potential barriers to the possible pathways just as we considered alternative goals for the aspiring professional athlete. A child that wants to be a professional basketball player need not be discouraged from this goal, but it may be helpful to help the child identify potential barriers to such a goal and potential alternative goals that can be pursued if this dream does not become a reality. Identifying barriers allow us to consider alternative pathways or detail strategies to overcome barriers. This will be critical in nurturing hope, as low hope people may be still focused on the potential for failure and demonstrate reluctance to continue down the pathway to hope. Focusing on barriers can also decrease willpower. Thus, we need to consider taking time to capitalize on the power of imagining success. Alternatively, sometimes a goal, even if unattainable, requires enough steps toward that goal that hope can rise. Professional sports careers often require success in high school sports and success in college sports. Success in sports requires good enough grades to get scholarships or at least avoid detention! Good grades become goal attainment that increase hope even if the ultimate goal is not achieved yet.

Stage 3 (Future Memories): Once we have identified viable pathways, it is important to reinvigorate willpower. We suggest a focus on the power of imagination by creating future memories. In this stage, the individual will reflect on how success will feel, consider how they will be impacted, how they will behave, or how others around them will be impacted by their success. In this stage, the individual creates a realistic image of success. Karianne told us that during chemotherapy she would regularly imagine what she would feel like when the cancer was gone. She needed to imagine it before she could believe that it could happen. This process of creating future memories serves to reinforce mental energy (agency). As the individual approximates the desirable goal, their agency and pathways thinking should be elevated reflecting higher hope. Furthermore, successful goal attainment (even with smaller steps toward a larger goal) allows the now hopeful individual to pursue related goals and further develop a trail style of hope.

Gary Smalley and John Trent in *The Blessing* talk about picturing a special future for your children. Helping children think about what they might be when they grow up, how they might be able to impact the world or serve others, and how special that future can be frames the future for those kids. In Camp HOPE America, we do the same thing. With the campfire glowing and kids in a safe and inspired place, we often ask them about their dreams. Once children share their dreams of what they want to do when they grow up, we talk with everyone about how they can get there. But imagining it first, is the future memories stage of nurturing hope. If we can dream it, we can do it. If we cannot imagine it, it is hard for it to ever become a reality.

Bessel van der Kolk tells the story of Noam whose school was near the towers in New York City on 9/11. Noam saw the first plane slam into the tower and was able to feel heat through the classroom window. The next day, Noam drew what he had witnessed including seeing people jumping to their death. And he drew something at the bottom of the towers. It was a trampoline. Noam said the next time the people would have to jump this would keep them safe.

Noam experienced terrible trauma—something he had no control over—but he had a supportive family and a creative imagination that prevented him from experiencing PTSD. He felt and saw things no child should ever see but because he never lost his ability to imagine or think about creating a different future—he was able to move forward with his life. Bessel van der Kolk's story illustrates a crucial connection between the trauma research and hope research.

Trauma is about the loss of imagination. Hopelessness is about the loss of imagination. Trauma can cause damage when someone ends up at the bottom of the Hope Continuum—apathy—where they have no control over goals or pathways in life-threatening situation. Imagination gave Noam the ability to imagine a different future in a 9/11 situation and create a goal and a pathway to help it become a reality—this is high hope. High hope saved Noam from the damage of an unimaginable experience.

When someone is not able to learn anything from a painful, helpless experience, they begin to experience damage from trauma. You cannot live in the past and the future. If you get stuck in the pain of the past, your hope will be very low. If there is no ability to imagine alternative futures for yourself or someone you care for, trauma starts to do damage to the mind and the body. If you are able to choose to live in the future, imagining that different future, you have a pathway to hope. Imagination—picturing future memories—is a crucial step toward hope.

Stage 4 (Hope Begets Hope): At this point, both willpower and pathways thinking should be elevated reflecting the idea of hope. An increase in willpower will allow us to fine tune pathways or consider alternative pathways. Likewise, success in pathway pursuit will increase our willpower. Because hope begets hope, we now can begin to see that other goals are possible and we have the power to make it so. Start with small goals if you need to. Small goals will inspire bigger goals later.

Hope as a Social Gift

The late Professor Dennis Saleebey once described hope in the practice of social work as "a process where sometimes we have to lend hope to others until they can find it for themselves." In this context, hope is very much a social gift we can give to each other. Once you have hope, you can give it to others in every social interaction. Emeka talked about needing to borrow hope from others early in his journey. To the extent this is true, it should challenge us to be more intentional in the way we interact. To the extent this is true, it should challenge us to be more intentional in the way we interact with others and what we say when they need us to lend them hope.

Another way to nurture hope is to consider our hope models. These can be leaders we admire, adult role models in our lives, or even movies or books that inspire us. Let's take a few moments to consider these models and the social gift of hope they provide to us.

Hope Inspired Leaders: Research has shown that transformational leaders produce hope in those who follow their vision. Think of a leader you admire for a few moments and consider the characteristics you admire most. Now, list three words that describe this person. Research on thousands of subjects using this technique has found that hope was among the top 10 characteristics listed about an admirable leader. In Camp HOPE America, we use an evidence-based curriculum that always features biographical characters that were or are transformational leaders. Because the children we work with are all survivors of severe trauma and abuse, we always focus on leaders that grew up with profound trauma and overcome it to become inspirational leaders. In recent years, this has included author Maya Angelou, football player Michael Oher, Secretary of Education John King, Jr., Cesar Chavez, Olympic swimmer Yusra Mardini, Olympic athelete Jim Thorpe, Holocaust author Anne Frank, and many others. We will look at how we use them to inspire in the next chapter. Find a few hope-inspired leaders of your own and read about their lives as you are working through this book.

Adult Hope Model: Research on child resilience points to one common factor in helping children overcome adversity. Namely, children need at least one positive adult role model in their lives. Children need to learn and be affirmed that they are valued and matter. We would argue that as adults we need to re-learn and re-affirm this important lesson throughout our lives. The importance of being valued, is that— for the future to exist, for hope to exist—we need to know we are worthy of its gift. In Casey's book, *Cheering for the Children*, he called them "cheerleaders." Others call them mentors. But more importantly than any of those names, children need an adult role model living with high hope, not just a role model.

Take a minute to think of the one adult role model in your life who made all the difference in how you faced and overcame adversity at some point in your life. Chan had a middle school teacher come into his life at one of his darkest times. His middle school teacher helped him think about ways to a special future and reminded him of his value and worth. We will hear more of Chan's story later. For Casey, it was more complicated. His sometimes-abusive father was also his role model. He was affirming, encouraging, and supportive much of the time but also rage-filled, abusive, and irrational at other times. But when he played a positive role, he was helping Casey imagine a special future. He mitigated the very trauma he caused with his modeling of affirmation. As you think about your positive adult models, consider how they influenced your life in terms of goals, pathways, and agency. It is worth noting that researchers take this social gift provided by the adult model further and suggest the experience of gratitude you likely feel toward your role models is a significant predictor of your well-being. Even as you reflect on one role model, practice being thankful (gratitude) for the powerful role that positive adult played even if it was for only a season in your life. We saw earlier how survivors found hope in the process of practicing gratitude. This works for everyone.

Hope Movies, Songs, Books: We like asking students this question, "What movie most reflects hope in your opinion?" We both really enjoy watching movies so some of the ones they choose, we've seen: *Good Will Hunting, Shawshank Redemption, Blind Side,* etc. You can feel the positive energy as they call out the movies. If a student is particularly shy, we will stop and ask, "What was it about the movie that you liked?" We'll continue to probe with questions and clarifications even if we've seen the movie. Our singular purpose in this inquiry is to watch willpower flourish. Movies, books, and songs inspire us and can be a wonderful source as we attempt to nurture hope. This is especially true when we are facing adversity or feel mentally fatigued after days on the phone with AT&T.

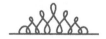

Chapter 17

Teaching to the Test
(aka Studying the Answers)

"We want to give every person hope. We must give hope, always hope."
—Mother Theresa

Carrie

Carrie grew up in a home with child abuse and domestic violence. Her dad began molesting her at a young age. It was all she knew. When she was 11 years old, she connected with a "boy" on Facebook who said he wanted to meet her. The next Saturday she went to a shopping mall in east San Diego County and met Aaron. He said he was 16 but he was 19 years old. She told him what she was living with at home and he said he would take care of her if she "ran away" with him. Weeks later, she moved into an apartment with him less than 10 miles from where her parents lived. They reported her as missing and even held a press conference with local law enforcement. But Carrie was not going home to be molested by her father again. She believed she had found a new home with a man who would love, respect, and protect her. She would later say the first three months were the "happiest of my life." The happy days ended when she arrived home one afternoon from a visit to 7-11

164

and there were three men with Aaron in the apartment. He said he owed them money and she needed to have sex with them or they would kill him. The gang rape that afternoon would send her into a downward spiral that would produce sexually transmitted diseases, methamphetamine addiction, severe depression, and suicidal ideation within a matter of months—at the age of 12.

Carrie lived in seven different stables between age 12 and 17. She had sex with thousands of men—some were kind, some were violent. She was bought and sold for five years like an animal. She would later say she felt like she "lost her humanness." But a caring social worker reached out to her in her darkest moment after years of unimaginable terror, abuse, and addiction and offered her a pathway out of commercial sex trafficking. Carrie took it and continues to navigate her goals and her pathways as she struggles to find her way to a college degree from San Diego State University and a career as a social worker for other trafficking victims. She has gone public with her story in documentaries and regularly speaks to teenagers about the allure of predators when girls and boys are trapped in homes with abuse.

When you ask Carrie, how she got out, you will eventually hear every element of hope. Her language does not exactly track the science but it is stunningly close. Carrie's life was saved because of advocates and social workers that knew she needed hope above all else. She needed to be able to see her life in the future as different than it was in the present. She needed to believe that her dreams could come true. She needed to know that caring people would cheer for her all the way to successful navigation of her new pathways.

In almost any discussion about education in the United States today, all you need to do to enliven a dry and boring discussion is to raise the issue of "teaching to the test." When this topic comes up in circles of educators, sides form, highly skilled and experienced educators take sides, and the tension rises in the room in nanoseconds. Some argue that teaching to the test does not help children learn the critical thinking necessary to then apply what is learned in real life environments. They say all you are doing really is studying the answers to the examination when you "teach to the test." This means children know the answers when they take the exam but they have not really learned anything.

Others argue that teaching to the test helps students perform better on standardized tests because they are learning the material that they will be tested on by the examiners. Therefore, some argue that teaching the answers makes sense because now children can pursue higher achievement levels with greater educational options available to all those who do well on the examinations. Once fully understood, the science of hope should never inspire this debate.

Our goal in everything we do should be to give hope, to cause it to rise in our lives and the lives of those we care about. When it comes to the science, **teaching to the test works**, educates, and inspires children and adults toward a brighter future. When it comes to the science, our research confirms you should ALWAYS "teach to the test" and help children know the answers.

If hope is transformational in our lives, and if nothing is more predictive of long-term success in life than rising Hope scores, there should be no debate about teaching to the test. We just need to know what to teach. What will raise hope to help us mitigate the risk of cancer or heart disease, to survive natural disasters, to overcome trauma, to improve self-care choices in our lives? What will change the endings for those we might be helping in non-profit organizations working with the homeless, the abused, the traumatized, and the marginalized? There are many ways to approach teaching to the test, but let's look at lessons we can learn from Carrie and our nationally-recognized Camp HOPE America work with children and teens who have experienced physical abuse, sexual abuse, and witnessed terrifying violence. This chapter takes the curriculum of our work with abused kids but presents it in a way so that every reader—whether you have trauma or major challenges in your life or not can apply it. In the Camp HOPE world, it has produced publishable research results including increased hope. It will work for you as well. Since this is based on the validated Children's Hope Scale with minor changes to include more measurement of agency (motivation), we will use the elements of hope from that scale but any adult will benefit as well!

Your Hope score will rise if you can say all these things are true about you most or all of the time:

- I have friends that really care about me
- I am part of a group of people that really care about each other (community)
- I like to encourage and support others
- Others accept me just the way I am
- Even when bad things happen to me, I still feel hopeful about the future
- I think I will achieve my dreams

To help operationalize these statements in your life, we want you to memorize these five statements:

- **My Dreams Can Come True**
- **Good Friends Can Help Light My Path**
- **I Am Resilient**
- **My Future Can Be Brighter Than My Past**
- **My Light Can Inspire Others**

Seriously, close your eyes and memorize them! Let's take them one at a time and use a few biographical hope heroes to help you remember and contextualize these powerful hope statements in your own life.

My Dreams Can Come True

John King: "Public school teachers are the reason I am alive. They're the reason why I became a teacher. They gave me hope about what is possible and could be possible for me."

John King was raised in Brooklyn, New York. Sadly, his parents died when he was only twelve years old. After that, John began acting out in school. He skipped class and even got kicked out of school! It must have been hard for John to keep believing in his dreams when he felt like the people that were supposed to support him either couldn't or wouldn't.

But one person, a teacher named Alan Osterweil, helped John see that the world was bigger than just his neighborhood. No matter where John came from, his dreams still mattered. Slowly, John began to move past his anger and take responsibility for his future.

With hard work, John was admitted into Harvard. He dreamed of becoming a teacher to help inspire kids who had difficult childhoods just like his. And you know what? John exceeded his dreams! After years of teaching, John became the Secretary of Education in the Obama Administration and oversaw all the teachers in the United States.

When John started to believe that his dreams mattered and that he could achieve them, his life turned around for the better. John King's dreams came true and yours can too.

John King's story is a great one. His mom died of early Parkinson's when he was 8. His father died of a heart attack when he was 12. His trauma led to rage which led to acting out in school, defying his teachers, and eventually getting expelled. He experienced logical, normal emotions and reactions to an abnormal situation. John lost willpower and waypower. As hope declined in his life, he descended the Hope Continuum from Hope to Rage and even, at times, all the way to Despair and Apathy.

Let's review his story. What was John King's dream? To be a teacher. What made it hard for him to focus on his dream and how to get there? The death of both his parents and poor decisions he made because of rage and despair. What helped him realize his dream could still come true? A caring teacher/friend. What steps did he have to take to get back on a pathway to his dream? What is one dream you have in your life? What might get you off your pathway? What steps do you need to take to get back on your pathway?

We saw John King's journey through Hope, Rage, Despair, and even Apathy and then the pathway back to Hope. No shame or blame for John King. He reacted normally to a stunningly traumatic set of circumstances and then, whether he knew it or not, the science of Hope gave him a road back to his dreams coming true. The statement became true in his life: "My dreams can come true." Say it again. Say it out loud. "My dreams can come true."

Good Friends Can Help Light My Path
Michael Oher: "I have been very blessed to have some great mentors and friends in my life. I know they all made a difference—some big and some small—but every positive thing had an impact and helped me get to a place where I was able to achieve my potential."

Michael Oher was born in 1986 in Tennessee. His mother used drugs and his father was in and out of prison throughout most of Michael's childhood. Because of his parents' poor decisions, Michael was placed into foster care when he was seven. He lived with lots of different families and attended eleven schools before he even reached the 9th grade. In one year alone, Michael missed fifty days of school because of rage, despair, and even apathy. He often got to a point where he really did not care about anything anymore.

But Michael did still have a dream of playing professional football. Michael's mentor, Tony Henderson, helped him get involved in sports even as he was on the verge of dropping out of school. Tony helped Michael get into a new school called Briarwood even though his grade point average was 0.6. At Briarwood, Michael became friends with a family that ended up adopting Michael and cheering for him at every single game.

To play in the NFL, Michael would first need to get into college so that he could play college football. With a lot of hard work (and with the support of others), Michael was accepted into the University of Mississippi where he continued to play football. After college, Michael went on to play football in the NFL. Have you heard of the movie The Blind Side? That movie is about Michael's life. Michael didn't achieve his dreams alone -- the support of friends and mentors lit Michael's path to the NFL.

Michael Oher is a great example of a traumatized, troubled child, who later became homeless as a teen, but found his way through teachers and other adults that befriended him, came alongside, and helped him find his pathway in life. He went on from the University of Mississippi to play for the Baltimore Ravens, after being drafted in 2009. He has also played for the Tennessee Titans and the Carolina Panthers.

Let's look at a few questions. Michael couldn't count on his family to believe in him. What might he have been feeling when he finally found people who believed in him? Who is one person outside of your immediate family that has believed in you as a child or as an adult? What were you able to accomplish because that person believed in you?

As we have seen, the journey is not linear out of tough times. Recently, Michael Oher was arrested for assaulting an Uber driver in Nashville, Tennessee. Oher ended up pleading guilty and taking responsibility though there was enough blame to go around with the driver ending up right in his face during an argument. Michael had been drinking which also likely clouded his judgement. When we make mistakes because of poor choices, what is usually the best path forward?

The truth about Michael Oher? As a child and as an adult, he needed friends that really cared about him—both peers and adults. Michael needed to and still needs to feel like he belongs to a group, a community, that cares about each other. Without those pieces at key moments in his life, Michael's hope plummeted and his decisions were self-destructive and unhealthy. With those pieces in his life, his level of hope rose and his decisions got healthier.

Every child and adult with high hope needs friends that really care about them and they need to be part of a community of caring human beings—both are key components in the science of hope. Teaching children and reminding adults how to pick good friends and discern between people that only take from them versus good friends that are interested in their well-being is foundational to everything else.

The second element is a perception that we are part of a community that really cares about us. A child may get this from a youth group at church, a soccer team, or a hundred other opportunities but every parent should be having this conversation with their kids. Every one of us should be evaluating this in our own lives. "Do you feel like you are part of a group that really cares about each other?" "Do you feel like your co-workers really care about each other?" "What could you do to help your friends show they care about each other?" As an adult, we might get this from colleagues at work, a social group we belong to, or even a close-knit family. It is the language of hope. It is teaching to the test on agency/motivation—the power of friends to encourage us in setting and achieving our goals. Ready to say it out loud? "Good friends can help light my path."

I am Resilient

Yusra Mardini: "Never give up."

Yusra grew up in Syria. From a very early age, Yusra was a powerful swimmer. Unfortunately, war broke out in Yusra's country, destroying her home and many others. To stay safe, Yusra and her sister decided to leave the country. Because of the war, Yusra had to put her Olympic dreams on hold. Her broken dreams were hard to process and she had few to talk to about them.

Yusra and her sister decided to escape Syria by boat. They joined many others fleeing war-torn Syria. Halfway through the journey across the Aegean Sea, their boat began to fill with water. No one had life vests. There were 20 people in a boat designed for six people and 17 of the 20 did not know how to swim. It was a recipe for disaster and profound loss of life. No food and no motor and only Yusra, her sister, and one other woman knew how to swim. Yusra got out of the boat in the middle of the Aegean Sea and swam alongside the boat, through white caps, for more than three hours. She pushed the boat for over three hours until they reached the shore of Greece. Yusra saved her sister and twenty other people on the boat. The media soon dubbed her "Courage Girl."

After the boat safely reached land, she made her way to Germany where she could swim again. A swim coach in Germany told her if she worked hard she might be able to compete in the Olympics by 2020, but it was too late for 2016 with the Olympics only months away. But Yusra began training for the Olympics as a member of the first Refugee Olympic Athletes Team and she qualified to compete in the 2016 Olympic Games in Rio. Her whole team was made up of people who had left their countries because of wars, too! Her team competed in the summer 2016 Olympics in Rio de Janeiro when she was only 18 years old and she even won her first heat against swimmers that been training for years.

Yusra has now set her sights on the 2020 Olympics in Tokyo, Japan. In between her training sessions, she spends her time using her voice to help other refugees. Yusra's most important message has become "Never give up."

Someone who is resilient can overcome and move past difficult things that happen to them. What did Yusra have to overcome to achieve her dream of being in the Olympics? What is one thing that you have had to overcome or that you are trying to overcome so that you can pursue your dreams? Yusra chose to encourage and help other refugees. Who can you encourage today? What does it look like (and feel like) to cheer for others and remind them to never give up on their goals and dreams? Yusra's resilience can be inspiring to all of us.

Resilience is about overcoming obstacles, bouncing back after setbacks, and still staying focused on your goals. It correlates to key components of hope: "I can think of many ways to solve a problem/Even when bad things happen, I still feel hopeful about the future." Time to say it out loud, "I am resilient." Louder, please.

My Future Can Be Brighter Than My Past

Maya Angelou: "My mission in life is not merely to survive, but to thrive."

Maya Angelou is remembered as a well-known American author and civil rights activist. But Maya had a rocky path to get there. Maya was raped by her mother's boyfriend when she was 8 years old. Her rapist was prosecuted and convicted but given only one day in jail. The judge essentially blamed Maya for the rape. Days later, he was murdered though his murderer was never caught. Maya blamed herself for his death, thinking because she had told about the rape that he ended up dead. She stopped talking after the murder of her rapist and did not speak again until she was 13 years old. Before and after the rape, Maya lived in a home filled with abuse and her parents split up when she was young. She and her brother were raised by their grandmother. Not having a stable childhood was very hard for Maya and her brother.

Even though she didn't talk for five years, Maya loved reading and writing. One of Maya's favorite teachers encouraged her to start reading aloud when she was 13 years old. Slowly but surely, by reading aloud, alone at first, Maya eventually found her voice.

Maya Angelou grew up to have a loud and important voice. She was awarded over fifty honorary college degrees in her lifetime. Some of Maya's most well-known stories discuss the bad experiences that she had as a child and how those experiences formed her into the woman and author that she ended up becoming.

Maya could have let her childhood hold her back from having a bright future, but she didn't. What did she need to let go of to move forward? What do you need to let go of so that you can become the person that you want to be? What would your attitude be like if you started believing that your future will be brighter than your past? Maya wrote poetry to help her envision her brighter future. What is something that you can do or say to yourself to remember that your future will be brighter than your past?

Maya Angelou wrote hundreds of poems and was a prolific book publisher. She was one of only two poets to ever speak at the Inauguration of a President. Maya

Angelou's poem "I Rise" adorns the wall of the Civil Rights Museum in Greensboro, North Carolina today. It is one worth reading over and over. Though more profound for women of color and the oppressed and the marginalized in our society, it has a message for everyone facing challenges from low hope.

Still I Rise
By Maya Angelou

You may write me down in history
With your bitter, twisted lies
You may trod me in the very dirt
But still, like dust, I'll rise.

Does my sassiness upset you?
Why are you beset with gloom?
'Cause I walk like I've got oil wells
Pumping in my living room.

Just like moons and like suns,
With the certainty of tides,
Just like hopes springing high,
Still I'll rise.

Did you want to see me broken?
Bowed head and lowered eyes?
Shoulders falling down like teardrops,
Weakened by my soulful cries.

Does my haughtiness offend you?
Don't you take it awful hard
'Cause I laugh like I've got gold mines
Diggin' in my own backyard.

You may shoot me with your words
You may cut me with your eyes,
You may kill me with your hatefulness,
But still, like air, I'll rise.

Does my sexiness upset you?
Does it come as a surprise
That I dance like I've got diamonds
At the meeting of my thighs?

Out of the huts of history's shame
I rise
Up from a past that's rooted in pain
I rise
I'm a black ocean, leaping and wide
Welling and swelling I bear in the tide

Leaving behind nights of terror and fear
I rise
Into a daybreak that's wondrously clear
I rise
Bringing the gifts that my ancestors gave,
I am the dream and the hope of the slave.
I rise
I rise
I rise.

Chanting it feels good for the soul. "I rise", "I rise", "I rise." Where are you now? In a Starbucks? In your living room? Chant it. We dare you. As you picture a brighter future and experience rising hope, let it out. That means you move your lips until sound comes out! I rise, I rise, I rise. And don't forget the main piece, *"My future can be brighter than my past."*

My Light Can Inspire Others

Jim Thorpe: "I am no more proud of my career as an athlete than I am of the fact that I am a direct descendant of that noble warrior [Chief Black Hawk]."

Jim Thorpe was born "Wa-Tho-Huk", which means "Bright Path." He had a twin brother, who he called his best friend, who died when he was 8 years old. Trying to protect him from the memories of his brother and fearing discrimination in America because of his Native American heritage, his parents changed his native name and sent him away from his home in Oklahoma to a boarding school in Kansas. Jim quickly realized he was looked down upon as a Native American boy at his boarding school. He was quickly branded as a "problem student" and struggled to find his way. Jim ran away from the boarding school and found his way back to Oklahoma to be with his family. His parents sent him away again to a new boarding school in Pennsylvania, believing it was his best chance to have a live different than theirs in rural Oklahoma.

At his new school, he discovered track and field sports along with football, basketball, and baseball. He was only 5'8" but he was a very talented athlete and worked harder than anyone else. He found coaches who believed in him and helped him to a pathway toward his dreams to play professional sports. After high school, he played minor league baseball for two summers before he decided that he wanted to try to qualify for the Olympics. The next year Jim Thorpe qualified for the U.S. Olympic Team in track and field. But even being picked for the Olympics he faced many critics who called him "the lazy Indian" and claimed (falsely) that he drank before he competed. The stereotypes he faced were ugly and powerful and Jim had to focus on his goals and dreams instead. He went on to win three gold medals at the Olympics in Stockholm, Sweden in 1912. Jim Thorpe always celebrated his Native American heritage even though he faced many stereotypes from people who were racist or discriminated against him. In 1913, he was wrongfully stripped of his Olympic gold medals because of accusations that he was not an amateur athlete, which was required at that time. Because he was paid a few dollars to play summer baseball before becoming an Olympian, they took away his gold medals!

Jim Thorpe's pain became his power though and he went on to play professional football, baseball, and basketball! What would it look like for your pain to become power? Jim Thorpe's life inspired thousands of other Native American children. What would your life look like if you were a hero that inspired others? What are some of your real-life abilities that you can use to encourage and support others like family members, siblings, or friends? What can you do to inspire others? Who is someone that inspires you to become the best version of yourself? What makes them so inspiring?

There is a Strength of Character Index connection to hope in the theme about our light inspiring others. It is gratitude and social intelligence. Hope-centered people learn the joy of encouraging and supporting others. Serving others, loving others, and reaching out to help others even when you are in a tough place brings hope and healing to the server. As we have seen, it gets you out of total self-centered, self-absorbed struggle and darkness and lets you see the world as others are experiencing it. It also brings in the notion that the choices you make are an example for others around you—for good or for bad. But when your decisions are healthy and hope-focused, others get inspired—their dreams can be ignited by your hope.

Jim Thorpe, "the Bright Path", is a great biographical character to help us think about stereotypes and the way stereotypes can keep us down until we realize we can choose our own path. He ignored the names people called him and focused on his own goals. Stereotyping is another form of victimization that so often piles onto other pain we have had in our lives from the death of loved one, bullying, poverty, or fear in our homes—the view that the "delinquents" will never amount to much or the angry child should be disciplined and shamed to cause them to make different choices in how they act. "You're nothing. Your nobody. You will never amount to anything. You are stupid. You are lazy. You are slow. You just aren't that bright. Don't pretend like you are better than me." But as we speak different words to ourselves or the hurting children around, all of us can begin to see that our overcoming can inspire others. Our refusal to be deterred from our goals can give others the courage to pursue their goals. Say it, "My light can inspire others." Say it again. Say it out loud, please. The people in the other room cannot hear you. We won't make you write it on the board. We are not shame-based. Just say it a few more times out loud!

Strength of Character is Power

We have talked about strength of character (traits) a number of times. Here are the core strengths we should all want to see increasing in our lives:

- Zest is an approach to life filled with excitement and energy
- Grit includes perseverance and passion for achieving long-term goals
- Self-Control refers to the capacity to regulate thoughts, feelings, and behaviors when they conflict with interpersonal goals
- Optimism is the expectation that the future holds positive possibilities and likelihood
- Gratitude is the appreciation for the benefits received from others with a desire to reciprocate with positive actions
- Social intelligence refers to awareness of the motives and the feelings of others
- Curiosity is the search for information for its own sake. Exploring a wide range of information when solving problems

Do you see how key theme statements connect directly to the science around hope and the character traits we need to cultivate?

Theme Statements	Validated Elements of Hope/Character
My Dreams Can Come True	I think I can achieve my dreams/Grit/Zest
Good Friends Can Help Light My Path	I have friends that really care about me/I am part of a group that cares about each other
I Am Resilient	Even when bad things happen to me, I am still hopeful about the future/Curiosity/Zest/Self-Control
My Future Can Be Brighter Than My Past	I think I can achieve my dreams/Optimism
My Light Can Inspire Others	I like to encourage and support others/Gratitude/Social Intelligence

It should come as no surprise that "teaching to the test" or "studying the answers" improves our outcomes in our lives around hope and character. You can do this in your own life, with your kids, or in an organization. If you want more hope, focus on the elements of hope to increase it in your life. If you want to advance character traits that will help you be more successful, focus on the elements of character.

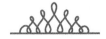

Chapter 18

Spirituality and Hope

"Pain is a traveling professor and it goes and knocks on everyone's door. The smartest people I know are the people who say, come in and don't leave until you have taught me what I need to know."
—Glennon Doyle Melton

Casey

I don't remember the first time I was afraid of my dad. It was early in my life. He would get angry and frustrated and it was always my fault if he was mad. He wasn't always mad though. He was kind and loving too. Maybe that's why it was confusing. I remember sometimes being happy when he was mad at my sisters or my brother. It wasn't me. And when he was nice it was the best.

My dad was all-powerful. He seemed to never make a mistake and I learned early not to question him or try to talk to him when he was mad. Many years later a therapist would ask me why I never told my dad how his anger and violence made me feel when I was a child. I got up and walked out of her office. I had to find a better therapist.

Dad didn't call it violence. He called it discipline. "Spare the rod and spoil the child." "Quit your crying or I will give you something to cry about." It always seemed like a stupid statement since I had something to cry about—that is why I was crying. But I learned not to cry. I learned not to show an ounce of emotion when he whipped me. The only emotion I remember was anger. I looked forward to when he calmed down and told me that it hurt him more than it hurt me, even though I thought that was horseshit. But I never would have said horseshit in my Dad's presence.

I remember many instances when my father held me down while my mom rubbed a bar of soap in my mouth and across my teeth and then made me swallow. I never said a swear word but there was clearly something I had said that was an unforgiveable sin. For the life of me, I cannot remember one thing I said that ever deserved the bar of soap in my mouth that made me gag and feel like I was choking.

He did to me what his father had done to him but not as bad. After my dad died in 2009, I learned that he was punched in the head by his father every day to be awakened when he was a child. "Wee Willie Wee, wake up," my grandfather would say before his fist greeted my dad's head. When my mom told me in 2010, she wondered out loud "It is amazing your father was as normal as he was given all those times he got hit in the head as a child." I asked her how it stopped. She said when my dad was 13 he woke up one day before my grandfather came in the room and as my grandfather approached my dad, now 6'0 tall, stood up to my grandfather, balled his fists and said, "If you ever hit me again, I will kill you." Then, my mom said matter of factly, "And you know…his father never hit him again." But I believe the damage was done.

My dad was bipolar, but I didn't know it. He was high energy sometimes and low energy at other times. He could go days without sleeping in the summer and get very moody in the fall. It worked well for a camp director at one of the largest Christian camps in America. He was a visionary, dreamer, big picture guy. He was an extrovert and he genuinely loved people. He was as winsome in a crowd or on a stage than any man I ever knew. And I saw all the great preachers and pastors in the country come through Mount Hermon Christian Conference Center in my growing up years. No one knew he was bipolar. He did not know either.

My dad's verbal, emotional, and physical abuse came and went during my growing up years. He ran hot in stressful situations, but at other times he was the game-playing, laughing, tickling, affirming, loving dad that I wanted. He abused my brother more than me, but I didn't know that until I was 50 years old. I never even saw him hit my brother when I was a kid. I didn't see him hit my sisters at all but not all abuse is physical and not all injuries are visible. I just kept telling myself that was the way all dads were and it was no big deal.

My dad wasn't my only abuser. My mom had her own trauma issues from her childhood and she too would engage in oddly unkind and abusive behavior—perhaps connected to *her own parents. I was bullied in elementary school for more than three years and told no one. I also was molested by a store clerk in a JC Penney store while my mom stood feet away. I did not make a sound and I told no one while it was happening. Thirty seconds later it was over and I stuffed it where I have always stuffed everything—deep inside my soul—for the last 40 years.*

By high school, I was white hot inside at times. I never hit a girl though and rarely let my rage out. I channeled it into school, student government, sports, and achievement. The greater my achievements the more praise I got from my dad. It was easy to figure out what got me the most positive attention from my dad.

When I was 17, my dad got fired from his job. I did not know why. Later, I found out he had raged at one too many of his subordinates and his irrational behavior due to his mental illness eventually was his undoing. Two months later, he had a nervous breakdown. During his psychotic break from reality, he tried to go find Richard Nixon in San Clemente, CA to demand that he repent for his sins and ask the American public for forgiveness. The Secret Service and a dear friend of my dad's in San Clemente intervened and my dad went to a psychiatric hospital—the jail kind. For weeks, he called our home collect in Northern California and raged over the phone that we had abandoned him and he was going to die in "jail." At night, my mom would lock herself in my bathroom and talk through the door about killing herself and just wanting to die. I did not attend high school for nearly two months during that crazy time. The kindness of caring teachers let me graduate from high school and allowed me to still attend Stanford University that Fall.

I lived out my rage and found my coping mechanisms in college—sex, alcohol, risky behavior—they all worked well. They were a solution to my problem. Eventually, I found my way back to my faith in God, but it was complicated. When you are abused as a child, you think God is like your abuser. Only many years later, after I went to counseling did I understand the depth of my distortion. I was talking to a therapist and made reference to my dad's death except I said, "When God died..." She caught it and, then with a look, caused me to realize what I had said. My dad was God to me—often mad at me, focused on my achievements, and always expecting me to earn my way out of my misconduct and sin.

When I became a dad myself, I determined never to even spank my kids. It was too dangerous for me to go down that road. By the grace of God, I never did. As a child and as an adult, I never knew anything about trauma or the impacts of trauma. Even as an adult, I had never heard of the ACE Study or the kinds of behaviors that often follow childhood abuse and the subsequent rage it can produce. Even in the hardest times, when the heaviness would set in and drag me into a dark place in life, I had no self-awareness. My rage worked during my 20 years as a prosecutor. Men, mostly, did bad things to women and children and I held them accountable—sent them to jail and prison—and everyone cheered for me. It was not until we started Camp HOPE, our program for abused kids in 2003, that I began to realize that my pain could become power. That I would help other kids understand why they felt the way they did and why there was a pathway to a better life, a hope-filled life.

Truth: I am a 5 on the ACE Scale even giving my parents the benefit of the doubt. I know they did the best they could but they left me with lifelong impacts from the choices they made. I am still on a journey. I believe my future can be brighter than my past and I believe I have the power to make it so. I believe the grace of God is sufficient for me and anything I have done to hurt myself or others. I am choosing hope, facing my fears, and my pain is slowly becoming power. I know nothing will separate me ever again from the love of God that I have experienced through so many years of my life where authenticity and honesty have not been my pathways.

This chapter is written for people of faith and those interested in spirituality. We have many friends who do not share our faith, have deeply held beliefs that differ from ours, or who describe themselves as atheists or agnostics. With a deep respect for those who do not share our Christian faith, we have included this chapter because most adults and children do believe in God. In most studies, well in excess of 90% of children and more than 85% of adults believe in God.

America has many faiths and belief systems. We need to be sensitive to those faith systems and beliefs in the lives of all those learning about the science of hope. This chapter is written primarily for those whose hope is connected to faith in God. But even if you don't share our faith, understanding the deep importance of spirituality to many will help you support friends, family members, co-workers, and others when they face pain and loss and try to find pathways to rising hope. It is also important for understanding the needs of trauma survivors.

Many trauma survivors have grown up in homes where faith has been used as a tool of abuse. Even those who share our faith don't know how to address the trauma or help them find a pathway to hope.

Most research has found that after a traumatic experience, and once the victim's immediate physical and medical needs are met, the next set of needs include spiritual care. The research around religious and spiritual coping shows strong and convincing relationships between psychological adjustment and physical health following trauma. Spirituality provides a belief system and sense of divine connectedness that helps give meaning to the traumatic experience and has been shown over and over to aid in the recovery process.

The importance of spirituality has been well-documented with victims of hurricanes, fires, tornadoes, violence, abuse, the death of a loved one, terrorist attacks, and other forms of trauma. But even outside the context of trauma, those who consider themselves spiritual or religious tend to be happier, healthier and more socially connected. Psychologist Sonja Lyubomirsky from the University of California, Riverside and author of *The How of Happiness* argues that we "…can no longer ignore the powerful influences of spirituality and religion on health and well-being. If nothing else, the statistics should compel them."

Hope is the Anchor of Our Souls

Beth and Casey loved vacationing with their kids when they were young. Houseboating was one of their favorite vacations. Houseboating is camping on a lake. They loved the summer adventures of houseboating at Lake Shasta and Lake Don Pedro in California and Lake Powell in Arizona. One year they were at Lake Powell with two other families when they got hit by a monsoon. It was a sunny, beautiful day in the morning. By afternoon, the dark clouds had arrived, but they never imagined what was next. At 2 PM, suddenly the wind picked up, growing in velocity to more than 50 miles an hour. The houseboat was tethered to the shore with ropes on each side and two stakes in the sand of the beach. They had not dropped anchor—never expecting what was about to happen. Within minutes, as torrential rains accompanied the wind, the houseboat was torn from the shore, dragging the stakes and ropes with it. Casey and his kids were out wakeboarding when the storm hit and he had to try to re-board the houseboat as it was pushed across the lake with white caps everywhere. He tied the ski boat up to the houseboat as the two vessels slammed together over and over—causing major damage to the fiberglass ski boat.

Once on board, he tried to start the two outboard engines on the houseboat only to find that one was swamped with water and would not run. At one point, he looked out and saw that the houseboat was headed toward a large rock outcropping that formed a small island. The children were crying and everyone was praying. The outcome seemed bad no matter what the possibilities. But Casey was able to start one engine and he maneuvered the houseboat away from the outcropping into the open lake. Within an hour, the monsoon passed, the sun came out, and everyone watched waterfalls streaming down the sandstone rock faces that blanket the shores of Lake Powell as a massive rainbow formed in the sky.

The terrifying experience is etched in the minds of everyone that was on the houseboat that day. Without the boat firmly anchored, the wind and the waves broke it free sending it adrift into perilous waters.

Our lives often end up adrift in perilous waters without an anchor. What is your anchor? We believe the evidence is compelling and our vision for this book is to help you figure out how to make hope your anchor. If you are reading this book and find yourself adrift and without focus, you need an anchor and hope is the most solid anchor you can find.

Writing a book is a personal, vulnerable, intimate experience. This book has been no exception as we have each shared our personal experiences with trauma, our struggle to overcome childhood abuse, and the pathways we have chosen as adults. We would be hiding part of our stories if we did not include the importance of spirituality in this book. Hope is the anchor of our souls. Human beings are designed for hope—to believe that the future can be better than the past and that we each have a role in making it so. As a species, we are naturally optimistic and goal-oriented, until trauma or pain or major life stress damages our ability to hope. Then, we must pursue rising hope if we are going to restore our ability to thrive in life. We mentioned early in the book that the Judeo-Christian tradition was the first time that hope was described as a virtue like faith and love.

Shane Lopez often asked audiences whether they thought hope came from the heart, the mind, or the soul. Those with spiritual faith saw the source as the soul. Those with a more scientific bent saw it coming from the mind if they believed in hope at all. Those with a secular but deep-felt belief in goal setting and pathways thinking often thought of it as a heart issue. Early on in this book we said we saw it as a little of each but spiritual people often feel it more deeply than others.

Author Samuel Coleridge in *Work Without Hope* says, "Hope, without an object, cannot live." We each need to find an object—a goal—to focus our hope on if we are to be people of high hope. For people with higher hope, the anchor in tough times is hope. Underneath the notion of hope however, must be a goal. For us as people of faith, hope is the anchor and the anchor is planted in our faith in God. It is perhaps the most spiritually accurate definition of hope and it acknowledges the infinite and the eternal. Dr. Martin Luther King, Jr. said, "We must accept finite disappointment, but never lose infinite hope." But irrespective of your faith beliefs, hope must have an object. You must have a goal that you are pursuing so that you can believe the goal will be accomplished and you have a role in making it so.

If the Gwinn Family houseboat had been anchored firmly during the monsoon, it would have moved back and forth, but it would not have ended up adrift in the middle of Lake Powell. If the whole family had known the anchor was set firmly, there would have been far less fear, anxiety, and panic. This is the spiritual truth for people of faith as well.

The Bible says that hope is the anchor of our souls. It is a fitting metaphor. What is going to keep your soul in the right place in the difficulties of life? In the worst storms of life, what will keep you from drifting into anxiety, fear, despair, anger, and resentment? Our research is consistent with the Biblical concept of hope as the anchor for our souls. When you are anchored to hope, you have the best chance to overcome difficulties and navigate challenges in your life. People of faith also have an advantage. No matter what you face, no matter how big the challenges, you can know that God is bigger than what you are facing. He is still on the throne. God still has a plan for your life no matter how bad the storm gets. People of faith can claim the promise of the Bible that God causes all things to work together for good for those how love Him.

The science supports the concept of hope as an anchor, however, even if you are not a person of faith. Hope, your focus on goals, agency, and pathways, can buffer traumatic and difficult times in your life. Laural, one of our hope heroes from early in the book, was molested by her biological father. Laural does not share our faith in God. But she did choose hope as her anchor—setting goals to process her pain, tell the truth about her struggles, and find people to come around her that cared about her and accepted her without shame or blame. She also set goals around helping others that helped her heal as she invested her life in hurting children who had experienced similar trauma. Laural describes "nature" as one of her grounding forces. She describes "hope" and "love" as her anchors in life. We honor and celebrate her powerful anchors.

As people of faith, we describe our beliefs differently from Laural but hope is a powerful anchor for everyone.

We Have This Hope…

Karianne received a devastating medical diagnosis. Many in her situation would be upset, but Karianne was anchored to hope. Emeka went through unimaginable loss when he was paralyzed and his emotions started pulling him toward discouragement, fear, and bitterness. But his inner voice said, "I am going to be OK. God has a plan for my life." What was happening? Emeka was trusting in the anchor of hope. After being paralyzed, his goals needed to change. Some around him probably felt pity, and even thought there was no way his dreams could come true now that he would spend his life in wheelchair. Many people would have given up, but high hope propelled him to say, "God has a way."

Maya Angelou suffered more trauma in her life than a human being should ever go through. But she kept her anchor down and stay focused on her goals and finding those pathways to her goals. Raped by her mom's boyfriend at 8 years old, she struggled to find hope. She stopped talking for five years. But a caring, loving teacher convinced her not to pull up her anchor.

When life seems unfair, when your dreams take longer to come true than you thought, don't give up on your anchor of hope. If you pull it up, you will drift as fast as a houseboat across Lake Powell in a monsoon. What will you drift toward? Emotionally, it won't be a rocky island. It will be anxiety, bitterness, self-pity, and discouragement. You may have doubts and negative self-talk can creep into your head, but your anchor needs to kick in. You need to change the tape playing in your head from the negative to the positive: "I know the answer is on the way. There are still goals that I can pursue even during this heartbreak. I know I can find a pathway to my goals."

If your low hope domain is finances, you are not alone. Most Americans live with a mountain of debt. We think there is no way out from 30 years of debt and creditors giving chase. But if you are anchored to hope, you can set a goal. "I want to get out of debt as soon as possible." Then, you can begin to look for pathways and friends that can motivate you toward the steps you need to take. What if your children have lost their way? Maybe they lost their way because of things you did or didn't do. First, you may need to let go of the shame and blame. You need to face the fears that every parent has about their children's future. Then, you need to start thinking about goals. What are your goals for your kids? How can you stay focused on those goals no matter what? The negative thoughts come, but you stay committed to helping your children achieve their goals. As parents, we look forward to our children growing up and moving out on their own, but we are still parents until the day we die. Your children are always your children, and helping them achieve their goals should never stop.

The Bible says faith is the "substance of things hoped for." True spiritual hope is not wishful thinking. It is something you hope for (a goal) with the faith (belief) that you can accomplish it. Hope is the precursor to faith. First, you hope (set a goal), then you choose faith (the motivation to believe your goal can be accomplished). The Jewish Bible picks up this same theme in talking about King David. In the Psalms, he was down and discouraged. He wrote in his poetry, "Why are you cast down my soul? Hope in the Lord." He had to consciously realize that his circumstances, challenging and difficult, had caused him to pull up his anchor. He drifted from one coping mechanism to another—like many of us do in life. But then he decided to put his anchor back down and plant it again in the God he believed in.

There are times in all our lives when it is hard to be hopeful. We give up on finding the job we want. We give up on finding the relationship we want. We stop working to be the person our spouse or family need us to be. If we plant our anchor in our circumstances, we will end up in trouble. At times in both of our lives, we have planted our hope in other people, and they have let us down. At times, we have chosen unhealthy coping mechanisms and they have failed us.

For each of us, we have had to make a choice again and again to put our hope in the God who created the heavens and the earth. And we have found, without exception, that when we squarely placed our hope in God, we were not disappointed. The Jewish Bible tells the story of Joseph, who was betrayed by his family, thrown into a pit in the ground, and left there to die. What was he tempted to feel and do? Anger, despair, and even apathy—giving up on his goals and his potential pathways. Does this sound familiar from the Hope Continuum? The natural response to unmet expectations. He did get out the pit only to be sold into slavery and then falsely accused of sexual assault and imprisoned. Understanding the science of hope, nobody could have blamed Joseph for rage when his expectations did not meet his nightmare of real experiences. It would have been a normal reaction to a very abnormal situation he was experiencing.

But Joseph kept waiting for God to have the final say. He determined that he would not pull up his anchor of hope. He still had goals and dreams. He knew his hope was in the right thing—his deep faith in God. He was convinced that the forces of darkness could not stop God's plan for his future. Eventually, he was vindicated, reinstated, and then promoted to one of the highest leadership positions in all of Egypt—a Jewish captive became the ruler of a Gentile country.

We love the phrase in the writings of the prophet Zechariah when he called the Jewish people, living in captivity, "prisoners of hope." Even in the darkest circumstances, they still focused on their goal of freedom. Zechariah was calling them to cling to hope even in the most impossible circumstances. They kept their eyes firmly on a goal that was not realized until generations later.

If hope is your anchor, you don't give up on your dreams no matter how big the obstacles or how many the enemies. Sickness or disease can seem like the end of you. But if you pursue a pathway to high hope, you will not need to live worried, stressed out, anxious, and resentful. Ultimately, your hope cannot be in the doctors, the drugs, or even the treatment plan. Your hope must be deeper.

We love the passage in the Bible where the story is told of Abraham and Sarah believing in a promise from God that they would have a baby. How old was Sarah when God promised them a baby? She was 80 years old. It was their dream to have a baby but it had not happened. It says in the Bible that "all reason for hope being gone, Abraham hoped on in faith." He planted his anchor in hope—based on faith in God's promise. It was a crazy idea. How can a woman have a baby at that age? But Abraham and Sarah planted their anchors. At nearly 100 years old, history records that Sarah gave birth. Abraham and Sarah waited 20 years for the promise (their goal) to be achieved.

Sometimes there is no logical reason to hope in such long-shot ideas. Joe Bellezzo's doctor friends made fun of him for choosing hope as the anchor of his soul. Dr. Jerome Groopman was told he would live with pain the rest of his life. Groopman planted his anchor in hope and believed he could get past a life a pain and disability and he did. Dr. Groopman's client, Barbara, focused her goals on life after death once she knew could not defeat her cancer. Karianne was told she had a cancer that was fatal in the majority of all similar cases. Karianne decided that God would not have allowed her cancer unless He was going to use it for her good. She chose to believe that God would bring to pass what He started when she was diagnosed with Grey Zone Lymphoma. She kept her anchor firmly planted and found a pathway to remission and healing.

Sometimes we need to keep our anchor set in hope on goals that don't come true quickly or easily. Just because our goals sometimes take longer than we are planning, does not mean they won't happen. We have to make a choice to believe that our future can be brighter than our past and persevere even if the ultimate result may depend on faith in God.

If you are a person of faith, you need this message. When God puts a calling on your heart, will you choose to believe it and make hope your anchor? What if people say you are crazy or what you are pursuing can never happen? Ask yourself this question when you are doubting and others don't support you. Did God put the promise in you or your critics? In the language of hope, is this goal something that you believe in passionately enough to stick with it even when it takes longer than you wanted it to take?

If hope is designed to be the anchor of our lives, then it makes sense that if you don't stay anchored to hope that you will drift. And it will slowly suck the dreams right out of you. You will wake up one day negative and even bitter. The great cosmic truth, however, is that the forces of hope that are for you are greater than the forces of rage, despair, and apathy that are against you. Higher hope has more power and produces better results in every arena of our lives than lower hope.

Re-Anchoring

Everyone does eventually pick things to anchor themselves to. The question is, what are you anchored to? Are you anchored to worry, stress, or bitterness? If you are, just as we have talked about re-goaling, you may need to "re-anchor." People can miss their purpose. They can end up with an anchor that they need to cut. Another houseboating story from the Gwinn Family is a great lesson in having the wrong anchor.

One year when the Gwinn's were house boating, they heard about a man who had purchased a brand-new Master Craft wakeboard boat. It was worth tens of thousands. He was towing it on Lake Powell one day behind his house boat and started to feel a great deal of drag. He looked back and saw no sign of the ski boat he had been towing for hours. Stunned, he rushed to the back of the house boat thinking the rope had come undone and the ski boat was floating somewhere behind them. When he got to the back of the boat, he found the rope pulling straight down into the water. He tried to pull it up and found enormous weight on the other end of the line. It took some time to figure out that the ski boat—his new ski boat—had sunk under the house boat. The drain plug must have come out from the floor of the boat and his incredibly expensive ski boat had become an anchor under the house boat—more than 75 feet below the surface of the water! He used his radio to call the Coast Guard and said, "I need help. My ski boat has sunk while still tied to my house boat." The Coast Guard said they would check on the options and get back to him. An hour later the radio crackled and the Coast Guard dispatcher said, "You only have one option." She paused. "Cut the rope." "Cut the rope?!" "I will lose my ski boat!" The reply: "We have other priorities with severe weather approaching Lake Powell." Then, the radio went dead. Imagine the moment as he went to get a knife and then sawed through the rope until his brand-new boat became detached from the rope and sank to the bottom of the lake.

Sometimes we end up with anchors in our lives due to our poor choices. The ACE Study articulated so many of those unhealthy choices we sometimes make earlier in the book. We have no choice but to cut the rope and let go of the wrong anchor. If you are anchored to anger, bitterness, or disbelief, you need to cut the rope. What if you are anchored to fear? We have seen the power of fear. But remember that fear only offers us three options, fight-flight-freeze. If you don't need one of these, then fear will not help you—cut the rope.

In Proverbs it says, "hope deferred makes the heart sick." We have already seen this when we looked at the enemies of hope. Hope not realized can literally make you sick. Sickness cannot defeat you unless you let it. When we are not hopeful, something is wrong on the inside. Living stressed and worried weakens our immune system as we saw earlier. If you want to live a healthier life, you need to keep your hope anchor down.

And even if you have a goal or a dream that cannot become a reality. You can choose to pick other goals. You can make a failed goal an excuse or your pathway to a brand-new goal.

Pain is Not the Enemy

Author Glennon Doyle Melton at the beginning of the chapter talked about pain as traveling professor. Glennon has written a great deal on the relationship between pain and spiritual growth. Athletes and members of the military like to say that pain is just weakness leaving the body. Anyone who has lived with chronic pain or survived acute injuries knows that is a lie. But pain can be a teacher. It can slow us down when we are moving too fast in life. It can cause us to realize our humanity when we are burning the candle at both ends. It can remind us of our frailty and humanity when we are tempted to think we are invincible. A broken heart can challenge us to love again. Deep loss can help us re-evaluate what truly matters in life. Writer Caroline Myss has put it this way: "We are not meant to stay wounded. We are supposed to move through our tragedies and challenges and to help each other move through the painful episodes of our lives. By remaining stuck in the power of our wounds, we block our own transformation. We overlook the greater gifts inherent in our wounds—the strengths to over them and the lessons that we are meant to receive through them. Wounds are the means through which we enter the hearts of other people. They are meant to teach us to become compassionate and wise."

Casey's pain gave him the power to hold Lance in his arms on a dirt road and tell him he was loved even while Lance threatened to kill him. Colette's pain in losing her husband caused her to realize how much she wanted to be loved again. Christian's pain, deep enough to make him consider suicide, makes him a great counselor for and mentor to other kids in pain. Karianne's cancer became her pathway to growth. Terrible, challenging, painful adversity in our lives does not just have to produce shortened lifespan, heart disease, drug and alcohol addiction, and depression. It can also be a pathway to growth.

Lance and the Power of Spiritual Truth

The book began with Lance running across a field on the last night of camp. Another story from this hurting boy's first week at camp helps us see the impact of spiritual truth and how hurting children may choose to find comfort in it.

Casey saw Lance for the first time on Monday when he arrived at camp. His trip from the group foster home to Lopez Lake in Arroyo Grande, CA was the first time he had ever left the Central Valley of California. He got out of the van with a look of indifference. His baby face, gentle affect, blonde hair, and blue eyes belied the rage that lived inside him. As the week unfolded, Casey learned more of his story. He grew up in a home with violence and abuse, dealing with multiple men in his mother's life after his father left. His mom's parental rights had been terminated after years of drugs and alcohol as she self-medicated her way through her own pain. Lance was placed in foster care and would travel through multiple homes as he acted out his rage—running away at times, fighting with his foster parents, and engaging in a variety of self-destructive behaviors. Group foster homes are the last resort for a child welfare system unable to mitigate the pain and anger in the lives of so many children and teens. But Lance seemed to flourish at camp. He loved the zip line, tubing on the lake, and the water park. His mood fluctuated dramatically from hour to hour but he was happy to be at camp most of the time.

The last full day of camp was Friday. The kids went to Avila Beach, a picturesque beach town about 30 minutes from Lopez Lake. It was 70 degrees and sunny as the staff relaxed with the kids on the sand at the beautiful juncture of the San Luis River and the Pacific Ocean. Lance seemed to love the beach. He had never seen it before or felt sand between his toes. His tent group stuck together most of the day and explored everything. But as everyone packed up for the bus ride back to camp, Casey saw Lance face down in the sand—burying his face with his arms at his sides. He was non-verbal and gave no indication he was aware of those around him even as the other kids packed up, yelled, and played all around him. Casey tried to talk to him but there was no response as he burrowed his face deeper into the sand.

Casey's son-in-law, Mike Johansen, grabbed some ice dumped from a water jug brought to the beach for the kids and placed ice cubes in both of Lance's hands. "Squeeze the ice", Mike whispered in Lance's ear. And Lance's hands closed—clear evidence that he was once again mentally present. "Lance, you have a choice to make," Casey found himself saying. If you want to ride with me and Mike back to camp, say "1." If you want to ride the bus with the rest of the kids, say "2." Not a sound came from Lance's mouth but slowly the hand at his side stretched out one finger. As the ice slowly melted in both hands, Lance lifted his head and asked, "What kind of car do you have?" "A Jeep Grand Cherokee," came Casey's reply. Assured his ride was nice, Lance rose to his feet and said, "Let's go."

Once in the Jeep, Casey offered Lance his iPhone and said he could pick whatever music he wanted to listen to on the ride back. Lance loved the opportunity to have some power over his life. He started and stopped a dozen songs before he settled on a Christian song entitled "Flawless" from MercyMe and listened intently to a song about redemption, forgiveness, and grace. The words resonated throughout the Jeep. "There's got to be more than going back and forth between what's right and what's wrong... Let me introduce you to amazing grace. No matter the bumps, no matter the bruises, no matter the scars still the truth is, the Cross has made you flawless..." Lance smiled to himself as he stared out the window and relaxed into the soft leather backseat of the Jeep. By the time they all got back to camp, Lance was talkative but calm. He would yet trigger again and run that night at camp and end up in a restraint situation with Casey. But spiritual truth and the loving, trauma-informed actions of Mike Johansen gave Lance another opportunity to feel loved and cared for during his week at camp.

The Five Stages of Dying and Hope

Elizabeth Kübler-Ross, in her groundbreaking book, *On Death and Dying: What the Dying Have to Teach Doctors, Nurses, Clergy, and Their Own Family*, delineated five stages of dying. First, there is denial. "This cannot be happening." "This must be a mistake." Second, comes anger. For the spiritual, this looks like, "God, how could you do this to me?" Third, Kübler-Ross said patients enter into the bargaining phase. For the spiritual, she said this includes promises to God (church attendance or devoting the rest of life to serving others). For the secular patient, it often includes negotiating with doctors for other treatments or experimental cures. The fourth stage of dying brings on depression for many. It is the realization that the inevitable has finally arrived. The final stage is acceptance. Kübler-Ross found that acceptance often still included an "illusory belief" in the possibility of a cure or miracle.

Kübler-Ross called this belief "hope." She wrote: "The hope that occasionally sneaks in [is] that this is just like a nightmare and not true; that they will wake up one morning to be told that the doctors are ready to try out a new drug which seems promising, that they will use it on him and that he may be the chosen, special patient...No matter what we call it, we found that all our patients maintained a little bit of it and were nourished by it in especially difficult times. They showed the greatest confidence in the doctors who allowed for such hope—realistic or not—and appreciated it when hope was offered in spite of bad news."

Jerome Groopman in *The Anatomy of Hope* rejects Kübler-Ross' definition of hope. We do as well. Groopman uses the story of one of his patients, Barbara Wilson, and her journey through terminal cancer to reflect on a deeper meaning and definition of hope that is consistent with our research. Groopman described Barbara Wilson's hope this way: "Barbara Wilson's unique calm and acceptance were present from the outset—not surrender but steady realism; she set the parameters on her care with a clear-eyed vision of what was possible, what made sense to her, how she wanted to live, when it was time to die. She seemed to be always in control, of herself and her circumstances, dictating her own terms. And she never relinquished a vision of the future, even when she knew she would be gone. Barbara did not cling to a desperate belief that I would arrive at the bedside with a cure from the laboratory just in the nick of time…The kind of hope she showed me was very different from what Kübler-Ross described. Barbara's hope was real and undying."

"In her case, it reflected the fact that she had found purpose and created meaning in her life through relationships with her loved ones, and with her God. Barbara did not dwell on the ineffable questions, 'Why me?' and 'Why now?' She saw death as a natural part of life." His story of Barbara Wilson is an excellent example of the significance of spirituality in the life of a terminally ill cancer patient with "undying" hope. Each example he gives of her choices pick up elements of the science of hope and let us see why Barbara's high hope gave her strength and calm even until the end.

President Bush and Divine Appointments

Spirituality also allows people of faith to believe in divine appointments and deeper meaning behind opportunities we are given in our lives. Divine appointments are moments that don't happen by accident and often help us find direction and meaning.

In 2002, Casey and his staff opened the nationally acclaimed San Diego Family Justice Center. It was the first framework of its kind in the country, as we saw earlier, to bring 25 agencies together under one roof to help victims of child abuse, sexual assault, domestic violence, elder abuse, and human trafficking. In 2003, Oprah Winfrey endorsed the model as Casey got to present it for two days on her show. In 2003, President George W. Bush created a national initiative to fund creation of 15 more Family Justice Centers modeled after San Diego. President Bush asked Casey to provide leadership to this effort in a personal meeting in the West Wing of the White House.

The special announcement by the President was held on October 8, 2003 in the East Room of the White House. More than 200 domestic violence and sexual assault professionals were invited for the President's announcement though few knew what the President would be announcing. Casey had been asked to be at the West Wing entrance to the White House at 1:30 PM that day while all other invited guests were to be at the East Wing entrance. At 1:30 PM, Casey was ushered into the West Wing into a room overlooking the Rose Garden. He was joined by Diane Stuart, the Director of the Office on Violence Against Women and a mom and her daughter, along with Colorado Senator Ben Nighthorse Campbell and the Postmaster General, Jack Porter. It was not clear at the time, but the President also announced the creation of a special stamp that day to help fund domestic violence shelters. The little girl from Colorado had won the art competition for design of the stamp.

After the President greeted the girl, the Senator, and the Postmaster General. He came over to Casey. First, the conversation focused on the Texas Rangers and the San Diego Padres. The President had been a minority owner in the Rangers before his election. Casey did not know exactly what was being announced that day, but the President said, "We are following your leadership, Casey." Casey said, "Mr. President, we are here to follow your leadership." "No, you are going to be in charge of this," said Bush. Casey did not know what "this" was!

Finally, the President said, "Well, there are 250 people waiting for us today and you're my date." He reached out to shake Casey's hand and Casey did not let go. "Mr. President, this is a divine appointment in my life today." President Bush pulled himself close to Casey while still shaking his hand and said, "This is a divine appointment for both of us, Casey. Let's go be faithful."

An hour later, President George Bush credited Casey as the founder of the Family Justice Center movement and authorized $20 million to begin creating Centers across the country where hope would be the watch word and survivors and their children would find safety, the opportunity to create new goals for their lives, and pathways to achieve those goals. Today, there are more than 130 Family Justice Centers in more than 43 states and 25 countries with many more being developed.

We both feel the opportunity to write this book is a divine appointment for us to share the science of hope. It is our prayer that we have been faithful and that many others will find hope to be the anchor of their souls.

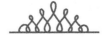

Chapter 19

Pursuing a Hope-Centered Life

*"**You** have brains in your head **you** have feet in your shoes. **You** can steer yourself any direction **you** choose."*

—Dr. Seuss

Chan

I grew up in a small farming community with a population under 1,000 and a graduating high school class of 21 students. We rented a small farmhouse when I was in the fourth grade having just moved back to NW Oklahoma from Tulsa, Oklahoma. This was the end of the Vietnam War and my parents were flower children "hippies" who protested the war and engaged in the drug culture. Beginning while I was in elementary school, my father became a drug dealer and had several hidden locations where he grew marijuana. My "job" was to help cultivate (planting and "topping"), harvest, and package the marijuana into ¼ to one ounce bags. My dad used to take me on drug sales that I now believe were his effort to reduce the chance of violence by buyers. As a small child who was already accumulating an ACE score (molested when I was four years old and physically abused by relative), I desperately wanted the approval and love of my father. Within a short time, I came to understand that our" family business" was illegal. I developed an intense fear of law enforcement. I became so terrified that the police would take my parents away that seeing a police officer would send me into a paralyzing fear. Each night I went to sleep in fear that the police were going to raid our house.

We lived in a very small community where the cliché that "everyone knows everybody" is absolutely true. We were the poorest family in the community, often living without household utilities (water, electricity, air conditioning for summer, heat for winter, phone). My childhood was filled with constant fear and shame. It wasn't long before I developed a belief that I was "less than" other children and as a result became embarrassed by my own name.

Despite this, or perhaps as a defense mechanism, I have always been good at building relationships, being known as a friendly, easy-going person. I was active in sports but never more than a marginal student in the classroom. Thinking back, I believe my ability to build relationships as a child was a survival strategy that I thought would buffer the fear and shame.

When I entered the seventh grade my parents got a loan to buy a small house in town. Moving from the rented farm, I now lived in a house that everyone would see. This "new" house had a leaky roof and a dirt floor basement that would flood at any rainstorm. At about this same time I was being bullied and tormented by one of the children in my class who now lived on the same block. I not only lived in fear and shame due to the "family business" but also in fear for my day-to-day physical and emotional safety from a bully.

Within a few months of moving into our house, my parents announced they were going to divorce—throwing my world into turmoil. My dad moved back to Tulsa with his girlfriend and had limited interaction with us. Of course, child support was non-existent. I believe my mother tried her best, but spent a brief time hospitalized for depression. She had dropped out of high school, and was able to get a job in the city 40 miles away. Perhaps the pressure was too much, as she just stopped coming home.

In the 7th grade, my life was in complete turmoil. My parents were gone, I only ate at school lunch or occasionally at a friend's house. Because we lived in a small town, I was convinced everyone knew what was happening. I was living in poverty and had become embarrassed of not only my situation, but of my life. I was ashamed of who I was. I didn't know what the science of hope was at the time but I look back and identify myself in the depths of despair.

There are two events that changed the course of my life.

The first event that happened highlights the importance of adults who nurture hope in a child's life. I had a science teacher, Gerry Walters, who was also the basketball coach for our middle school team. One day, as I was sitting on the gym bleachers, Gerry Walters came up to me, sat down next to me and put his arm around me. With his arm around *my shoulder, he leaned close for a long moment and said, "You are going to be alright, Chan." His simple act of authentic kindness showed me that I was a person of value—that I mattered.*

The second event happened at about the same time. I remember being home alone one night sitting in our dark house because the electricity was turned off. I was in such despair and felt so alone. I decided to get our gun and remember sitting for some time with the barrel under my chin. This is a flashbulb memory for me. I remember the look and feel of the couch. I can remember the feel of the gun in my hand. As I sat, I could see the dark living room—making out the television, lamps, and the floor. I can still feel the warmth of the dark summer evening and being alone with a gun under my chin. I thought about my options. I thought about the promise of, Gerry Walters, a caring man saying, "You are going to be alright, Chan." I knew I had to decide if I would be defined by my situation or if I could imagine a future as he had defined me. I was better than this, I was going to escape my poverty, trauma, and shame. My future would be better than my past.

It wasn't until later that a therapist helped me understand that my childhood safety and well-being were secondary to the needs of my parents. I have struggled because of my high ACE score. I have engaged in destructive behaviors and battled addiction. I suffer from anxiety, hypertension, high blood pressure, and still have many more days than not where my self-esteem is rocked by my past. During these times, I must work hard to overcome self-defeating thoughts and feelings of being "less than." I can see the science of hope at work in my day-to-day life. Most times, it is the positive relationships in my life that help me get through each day. Truly I am blessed, I have a loving wife of over 30 years, beautiful and healthy children and grandchildren, and an amazing professional career where my job is to study the science of hope.

For me, hope has become a personal journey. I can see how my life has been greatly impacted by the presence or lack of goals and pathways. My goals as a child kept me alive that night on a couch with the gun in my hand. I can see how hope is a precious gift and I was given it by a man with high hope who took the time to see me in that gymnasium. Our connectedness to others is so critical in our own ability to nurture hope—every achievement is based upon those who nurtured our willpower or serve as a pathway. For me, hope is the reason I'm alive today. The boy who was an 8 on the ACE Scale would one day marry, have a family, pursue a graduate education in psychology, and become a professor at the University of Oklahoma, and be able to talk with humility but clarity on how to live a hope-centered life.

One of the best books on nurturing hope is Dr. Seuss' "Oh the Places You'll Go!" It is filled with positive encouragement for a journey that is filled with ups and downs. It promises a journey that leads to sure success, except when it's doesn't. It is a fantastic story that reminds us that as we pursue our dreams, sometime things will work out as planned and sometimes they will not. However, several important issues need to be considered in this story. Hope is inside of you and pursuing your goals is in your power to control. Hope surely involves some level of risk and achieving your goals is not guaranteed. However, hope requires you to select pathways that are within your reach and to exert your willpower when pursuing your goals. It is not based upon luck or forces totally outside your control. It is about action. It is about intention. One of the most important ideas that is consistently found in research is that hope can be learned and must be nurtured because we have brains in our heads and feet in our shoes and we can steer ourselves anywhere we choose.

Living a hope-centered life is based upon your ability to (1) clearly define goals and set a vision for success, (2) identify pathways to goal attainment while considering workable solutions to possible barriers, and (3) the capability to focus your mental energy toward your selected pathways and problem-solving needs.

As we have described, the component of hope called willpower is perhaps the most difficult to put into motion and then sustain. You must be very intentional in how you dedicate mental energy to your road maps. How will you manage your willpower when you learn the pathway is wrong? How do you react when seemingly insurmountable barriers get in your way? One of the lessons from Dr. Seuss' "Oh the Places You'll Go" is that you almost habitually engage in the mental self-talk of "I can." The teacher that helped Chan move toward hope used to say, "Can't never did anything." This was a way of moving him away from his negative self-talk. This chapter is about making the choice to actively pursue a hope-centered life. You can apply the science of what we have learned to increase hope in yourself and be an active part of helping others.

Hope is an important protective force when we face common daily stressors (e.g. slow traffic as we drive to work, an inefficient barista at Starbucks, or AT&T Internet) but more importantly when we face life's big challenges. In times of high stress, hope allows us to identify and prioritize our valued goals, select the pathways to achieve these goals, and find the willpower to make our goals happen. With the help of a school teacher, Chan began the difficult journey toward his goals with the power of higher hope.

A Hope for Imperfect People!

Hope is the perfect answer for imperfect people. Living a hope-centered life is not simple or easy. It takes work. It takes honesty too. Each of us grew up with trauma and abuse. We have each chosen poor coping mechanisms in our lives at times. But we are moving beyond the shame and blame we could swim in every day, and choosing hope. Once you choose hope, then we must keep choosing it every day. Rising hope in your own life will have tremendous benefits to you and those around you. As we both began to apply the science, we saw how every aspect of our lives was impacted by hope. When goals are clear and highly valued, we are motivated to find pathways and solve problems to achieve our goals. In these pursuits, more often than not, we had people around us who became our pathways helping us overcome barriers or cheering us on, motivating us to face our fears with courage. Living a hope-centered life includes recognizing if you are a barrier or pathway to those around you.

Though the language is simple (goals, pathway, agency), practicing hope can be difficult if you are caught up in the drama of daily stress and especially if you are caught up in guilt and shame. You are imperfect, we all are. Consider forgiving yourself for whatever haunts your past. Shame and regret always look back and say, "What if..." Anxiety and stress trap us in the now with the voice in our head saying, "If only..." But hope looks forward and asks, "What can I do? What is one goal for today? One goal for the week? One goal for this next year?" Then, hope begins to identify the pathways (step by step) that I need to go down to move closer to accomplishing each of my goals. As you begin to find your way, you can help encourage others. We can be hope givers and we need hope givers in our lives.

We have been working to develop tools to help increase hope. The remaining parts of this chapter provide worksheets we have used in hope workshops, trainings, and retreats. These worksheets have been refined through feedback from participants (both individually and in groups) and if you lean in, work hard, be honest you will feel your hope rise.

Requirements for a Hope-Centered Life

The following basic steps are required for purposefully developing a hope-centered life:

1. **Understand the core tenets of hope:** Goals, Pathways, Agency. To pursue a hope-centered life, you must understand the basic principles outlined time and time again in this book. As you practice listening for and observing these tenants, you will begin to recognize hope in action.
2. **Use assessments to measure hope:** We advocate measuring hope and then teaching to the test. This means focusing on each concept in the Hope Scales

and creating practical ways to internalize them. Building pathways thinking, problem solving, and willpower will increase your self-confidence as you prepare to pursue your goals.

3. **Identify deficiencies** in your application of the core tenants of hope through self-reflection, observation of behaviors in self or in others, and listening to the narrative stories being told. With practice, you can begin to observe specific indicators of goal deficiencies, pathway deficiencies (including problem solving barriers), and willpower.

4. **Generate strategies** to increase goal setting, pathways development, and/or willpower to increase hope.

5. **Evaluate Progress:** Use hope assessments to assess changes in your pathways and willpower. You can use this information to refine your strategies as you begin to see hope rising.

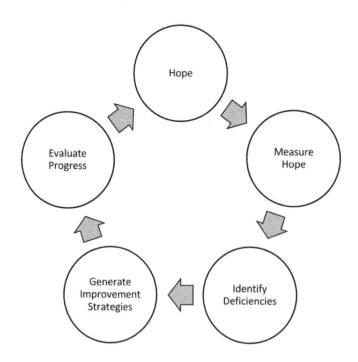

Using the Hope Worksheets to Nurture Hope

Based upon the science of hope, we have created a series of worksheets that illustrate our belief that the power to imagine yourself achieving your future goals is the cornerstone of hope. We have used these worksheets in countless hope workshops and trainings across the country. Additionally, these worksheets are being used in a variety of organizations. Some examples include social service agencies using them with clients, district attorneys' offices using them for staff development and attorney performance preview (as opposed to review), individuals using them for personal goal setting, businesses using them in employee training programs, and leadership academies using them for personal and professional coaching. We invite you to consider their application in your personal and professional life. We also invite you to adjust the wording and to add new questions as you deem necessary. We ask only that you give us feedback on their use and impact (positive or negative) so we can continue to improve the Worksheets.

Personal and Professional Goal Worksheet

This worksheet is intended to add detail and clarity to your goals. Those who are more hopeful will move through this worksheet with ease whereas less hopeful individuals will likely respond to this process with frustration and a focus on failure. It is important that obtaining the details to goals be pursued with patience and diligence. Do not rush through the worksheet. With each answer, spend time exploring more explanation and detail. The key to all these worksheets is to remember that imagination is the instrument of hope.

Goals

We provide space for three goals though more may be possible. Goals exist in all domains of our lives (i.e., family, work, leisure, education, etc.). Start this worksheet by simply listing up to three goals you want to achieve.

Take some time to consider some of the following details to add to your goals.

1. Approach (Positive) vs. Avoidance (Negative) Goals: Approach goals are those we want to attain whereas avoidance goals are those that we do not want to happen. An example of an avoidance goal would be, "I do not want to get arrested." Generally, hopeful individuals are more likely to set approach goals they want to pursue. Those lower in hope may be more inclined to describe avoidance goals. We touched on this earlier, but start where you feel most capable—whether your goals are negative or positive.

2. Goal difficulty: Some goals are relatively easy to attain and do not require much effort on our part. If a goal is going to be rather difficult to attain, we need to find specific opportunities to re-energize our willpower throughout our pathway journey. It is worth considering potential support elements early that we can call upon to assist us when times get tough.

3. Stretch vs. Mastery: Difficult goals may require us to stretch beyond our current skills and abilities. Stretch goals will require us to adapt to uncertainty and try out new pathways. Mastery goals are those that simply require us to deploy what we already possess. Hopeful individuals are generally likely to consider stretch goals as both a challenge and an opportunity for growth. Lower hope individuals will lean more toward goals that are within the confines of their abilities. Stretch goals may be seen as risky and more likely to result in failure. Gauge your willingness to fail. Failure is usually part of the journey for all of us in finding rising hope.

4. Time to completion: Is your goal based upon the short-term or long-term? Lower hope individuals are less likely to set long-term goals as they struggle to see engaging in the required pathways leading to success. It is important to understand that even hopeful people set short term goals. However, these short-term goals are likely seen as potential pathways to their longer-term goals. Pick whatever goals you can embrace right now.

5. Degree of Change Required: All goal pursuits require change. In organizational theory, change is considered in terms of first-order (small or low-level change) versus second-order change (large-scale change). For instance, pursuing a new job by moving to a new state far from your support network would be a second-order change.

6. Support Networks: When considering this section, it is worth thinking about the available support networks. Support networks can become important pathways in helping us achieve our goals and/or important to facilitating our willpower. Hope always thrives with friends, cheerleaders, relationships that encourage and build you up.

7. Beneficiaries: Who will directly and indirectly benefit when this goal is achieved? For instance, if my goal is to lose weight, I directly benefit through improved health and well-being. It is likely that my family will benefit as losing weight will give me more energy and they may be willing to support my pathway choices more effectively if they see benefits to their own lives from my goal achievement.

The final component of the personal and professional goal worksheet is to project how successful you will be in your journey.

A Note About False Hope

When considering this final section, take some time to understand how many of your goals are within your control to pursue (pathways). This is an important piece to nurturing hope. If you believe the outcome is solely dependent upon others, then we argue this is not hope. Pick other goals. We don't want you to aspire to be a better wishful thinker. When conducting hope workshops, we invariably get asked about false hope. We believe that if a person can set detailed, yet realistic goals and identify

Your Personal and Professional Goals Worksheet

Below write down three goals you set for yourself. These can be Personal Goals, Family Goals, and/or Professional Goals.

Goal 1: _____

Goal 2: _____

Goal 3: _____

Adding Detail to Your Goals

Specifics:	Goal 1	Goal 2	Goal 3
Approach vs. Avoidance:			
Degree of difficulty:			
Stretch vs. Mastery:			
Time to completion:			
Degree of change involved:			
Support Networks:			
Beneficiaries:			
Other Details:			

Overall, how successful do you think you will be in pursuing these goals?

1	2	3	4	5	6
Not at all successful	A little successful	Somewhat successful	Moderately successful	Mostly successful	Very successful

Goal 1: _____   Goal 2: _____   Goal 3: _____

the necessary pathways, this is not false hope. On the other hand, if you are setting goals that ignore the obstacles or pretend you have control over things you do not, this is false hope.

Hope Worksheet—Instructions

This worksheet is intended to add detail and clarity to your pathways and agency. Those who are more hopeful will move through this worksheet with ease whereas less hopeful individuals will likely respond to this process with frustration and a focus on failure. It is important that you focus on the details of the goals—taking the time to identify them with patience and diligence. Do not rush through the worksheet. With each answer, spend time exploring more explanation and detail. The key to all these worksheets is to remember that imagination is the instrument of hope. Imagine your life differently if you can achieve your goals. What will it look like? Feel like? Be like? You should notice the ebb and flow of pathways and willpower focus as you move through the worksheet.

As you review the hope worksheet below, some explanation is useful.

Item 1: Do not rush through this part of the worksheet. It is worth exploring each goal in terms of specific details, short term vs. long term, etc. The personal and professional goal worksheet may be useful in preparing for the full hope worksheet. A low hope person may struggle with describing specific details of a goal and might need help from a higher hope person. Don't be afraid to ask someone for help that seems to have higher hope in their life than you do.

Item 2: A person who does not desire the goal will struggle to complete the worksheet. It is important that the goal is desired by the person completing the worksheet. Finding a goal, no matter how small is often a great place to start if you are a low hope person.

Item 3: This item can help clarify the goal. For example, is the motivation to the goal intrinsic or extrinsic? Is it coming from within? Or is some outside force or person inspiring the goal? Goal motivation may start externally but sooner or later it must become internal. Intrinsic motivation is more likely to sustain you in the presence of barriers and adversity.

Item 4: After describing the goal, it is worth spending time relishing what success will feel like. This item is intended to reinforce willpower.

Item 5, 6, 7, & 8: Lower hope individuals will possibly struggle with these items. Don't be discouraged if you find yourself in that place. After considering the potential barriers, your willpower may be lower. Therefore, item 7 is intended to re-invigorate you to complete item 8.

Item 9: It is often helpful to break a goal into sub-goals or benchmarks. Sub-goals can also serve to help us determine if we are on the right pathway to our goals. Finally, breaking the goal into sub-goals helps you to connect the future to the present—seeing how the small steps can get you to the goal eventually. Dream big, start small.

Item 10 & 11: These are intended to reinforce willpower and demonstrate the social resources available when pursuing our goals. You likely have far more resources available to you than you might think right now. It may take being honest with others in asking for help and it may take the time to find the right person to ask for help. But take it one step at a time.

Remember, imagination is the instrument of hope. You must see it before you can be it. You need to dream it before you can do it.

Hope Worksheet

1. **Describe your goal in as much detail as possible (Narrative)**
2. **How much do you desire this goal?** *A little Moderately A great amount*
3. **Describe why you want to achieve the goal. That is, describe what is motivating you.**
4. **Imagine you have just achieved your goal. Describe how you think you will feel in this future memory.**
5. **List the pathways (actions/strategies) you can use to achieve your goal.**

Pathway 1: ————————————————————————————
Pathway 2: ————————————————————————————
Pathway 3: ————————————————————————————

6. **Describe potential barriers for each pathway you listed.**

Pathway 1 Potential Barrier: ————————————————————
Pathway 2 Potential Barrier: ————————————————————
Pathway 3 Potential Barrier: ————————————————————

7. **Describe a time when you achieved a goal by overcoming barriers. That is, what were the barriers and how did you overcome them?**
8. **From points 5 & 6 above, choose the best pathway and describe how you will overcome the barriers to that pathway.**

9. **Describe benchmarks that you need to achieve to attain the goal. For example, what are two or three things that must be accomplished for you to attain your goal?**

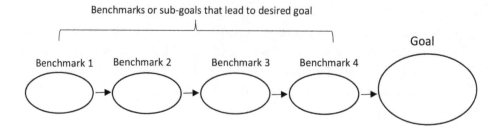

10. **Identify people and/or resources you can count on for support in pursuing your goal.**
11. **Describe something that motivates you (e.g., music, movie, person). Think of how you can use this inspiration to help you achieve your goal.**

Lean in. Don't give up. If you didn't do the worksheets, go back! You can do it!

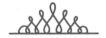

Chapter 20

The Hope-Centered Workplace

"You get the best efforts from others not by lighting a fire beneath them, but by building a fire within them."

—Bob Nelson

Harvey Weinstein's Victims

Angelina Jolie, Gwyneth Paltrow, Rose McGowan, Ashley Judd, Rosanna Arquette, Louisette Geiss, Heather Graham, Ambra Battilana Gutierrez, Tomi-Ann Roberts, Judith Godrèche, Katherine Kendall, Dawn Dunning, Lucia Evans, Laura Madden, Asia Argento, Lauren Sivan, Mira Sorvino, Emma de Caunes, Emily Nestor, Cara Delevingne, Jessica Barth, Kate Beckinsale, Zoë Brock, Louise Godbold, Liza Campbell, Romola Garai, Léa Seydoux, Claire Forlani, Florence Darel, and Sophie Dix. "Grabbed." "Masturbated." "Massaged." "Propositioned." "Cornered." "Kissed." "Overpowered." "Rubbed." "Exposed" "Chased." "Undressed." "Assaulted." "Manipulated." "Raped." "Scared." "Embarrassed." "Afraid." "Naked." "Bathtub." "Bathrobe." "Trapped." These are just a handful of the women that have come forward and a few of the words they have used about Harvey Weinstein that should not connect to the workplace or a healthy business relationship between an employer and an employee, contractor, or consultant.

As sexual harassment by men in American culture and particularly in the workplace has burst onto the public scene in the last year, it is difficult to find an easy way to talk about the notion of a hope-centered workplace. Our expectations are currently much lower than that. Can we keep men from raping women at work? Groping women at work? Demanding sex or sexual contact in return for a job?

But our focus here is on much loftier goals. Don't women and men deserve a workplace where they experience rising hope? How can we measure it in the workplace? How can we know if employees are experiencing it? How can we guide employers to aspire to a healthy, productive work environment through a hope centered work culture? How can you as an employee experience a high rate of hope in your work?

The Power of Rising Hope in the Workplace

Employees need hope today more than ever. In national studies over the last several years, Gallup finds that only 30 to 35% of American employees are "engaged" (fully invested and focused each day) at work. This "DIS-engagement" cost the U.S. economy roughly $450 billion every year. Shane Lopez found that only 13% of workers "love" their jobs. The problem is related to our own actions in the workplace, our work environments and it is fundamentally related to leadership.

Shane Lopez' research on worker satisfaction is sobering. He found only 13% of all people "love" their jobs. 87% are less than satisfied with their jobs. We need much higher levels of hope in workplaces. The problem is related to our own actions in the workplace, our work environments and it is related to leaders. First, the happiest workers have made their jobs into something they love. A job you love is made, not found. Second, most of them are in companies that have created cultures of hope, support, and community. Third, leaders in those companies are hopegivers. Leaders need to have hope to give hope to their employees. If you think about a supervisor or boss in your past that got the best out of you, the leader invariably challenged you to set goals and achieve them in a way that inspired you to set more goals and pursue even more pathways toward your goals irrespective of the obstacles.

Leadership Matters

The importance of the right leaders in companies is clear from the research. Gallup looked at this years ago by conducting telephone interviews with more than 10,000 people. They were interested in why people followed leaders. They found four major psychological needs that were met in the followers to inspire them to follow: Compassion; stability; trust; and hope. In return, if those needs were met, the followers responded with commitment, creativity, mutual trust, and engagement. A host of studies have confirmed the importance of rising hope in followers whether in a spiritual setting, an academic setting, or an employment setting. When employees have a boss that gives them hope, they are more excited about their job, more determined to stick with the job, and more likely to work hard at their job. As we saw earlier, hopeful employees are more innovative and productive than employees with low hope and they are more likely to stay with the company for the long-haul.

In contrast, employees know whether their employers are interested in their success and if they are not, they can even articulate it. During Casey's DEFCON journey with AT&T, he encountered a repair man that helped him find a creative way to get Internet while the Gwinn Family waited for the street to be torn up and the wiring to be replaced. His AT&T repairman, David, worked hard and came up with a short-term fix. Casey offered to give him a "tip." He declined for ethical reasons. Then, Casey offered to write a letter to his supervisor. The response of the employee? "It serves no purpose. No one at my office cares how well I do my job and no one will ever pay attention to a compliment I receive from a customer. They don't connect my performance with my future at the company." Perhaps not representative of all of AT&T, but still an interesting statement that no executive at any company should ever want to hear about an employee. The internally driven employee was a person of integrity finding his significance in his own goal setting and goal achievement, but his supervisors were not creating an environment where working for them was raising his level of hope.

The Gallup research found that the creative AT&T employee is really an anomaly in the absence of a healthy, positive, encouraging work environment. Of those followers who said their leader did not make them enthusiastic about the future, only 1% of them were committed and energized about their jobs. Workers with low hope are often a threat to themselves, co-workers, and the company. Sometimes they even drag down others and the research shows they are physically and mentally unhealthy more of the time. They also are not likely to stay with the company for more than two years on average. We both used to think that employees with short stays were a liability and we should not hire them. Now, we are questioning whether the problem was with the employee or with the companies they worked for.

At Alliance for HOPE International, we have correlated rising Hope scores with successful performance at work. Each year we measure the Hope scores of each employee and correlate those scores with their work performance. The result? Increased hope produces happier and more productive employees. Sinking Hope scores produce unhappier and less productive employees. Between 2017 and 2018, the average Hope score for the staff of Alliance for HOPE International rose from 54.06 to 57.25—giving strong evidence that the organization is giving hope to those it serves and to those that work there. The findings of the Alliance have been mirrored in a variety of work settings across the country. The Netherlands consistently ranks as one of the happiest places on earth with some of the most satisfied employees in government and private-sector jobs. It is no coincidence that they are also focusing on hope in their employee wellness programs and using many of the principles of positive psychology to motivate and inspire employees.

Jon Tunheim, the elected prosecutor in Thurston County, Washington, was the first DA in America to start measuring hope in his staff. They are measuring hope, job satisfaction, well-being, and turnover. Jon is also using the hope worksheet with his employees to better understand their personal and professional goals. Chan is currently even applying the notion of measuring hope in workers to an entire City under the banner "How Hopeful is Tulsa." They are measuring collective hope, individual hope, trust, connectedness, and basic needs (e.g. food, shelter, safety, and transportation). This is the kind of measuring that should be happening across the country.

Every employer in America should be measuring hope in the workplace. Social service and non-profit agencies working with trauma survivors and people in need should be increasing measurable hope in the lives of those they serve, but they should also be measuring it in their employees. If you cannot give, what you do not have, then every employer in the helping professions should be measuring hope to make sure their employees have it so they can give it!

But this should not simply be the case for non-profit organizations or the helping professions. Employees with higher hope will be more productive, more creative, and more loyal in every business environment. Companies without productive, creative, and loyal employees will rarely thrive for the long-haul—no matter what the service or the product they are selling. As we are learning more about hope-centered workplaces, the research is helping us understand these concepts on an even deeper level. One of the key concepts coming out of the research is the power of collective hope—rising hope in a group of people instead of simply rising hope in one person.

Collective Hope

If hope is such a powerful force for individuals, imagine the possibilities for collective hope. Collective hope is similar to individual hope in that it is based upon goals, pathways, and willpower. However, it includes the complexity of social influences necessary for shared values and beliefs. Collective hope requires the group to have a shared vision of the future (goals) and collectively agree on the strategies (pathways) for pursuing this vision along with a unified mental focus (willpower). As we saw at the beginning of the book, collective hope (shared belief in goals and pathways) among the staff members at the Sharp Hospital Emergency Department was what created a culture of hope.

The San Diego Family Justice Center

Early in the book we looked at Ellen's story and how she wanted and needed a "whole person care" model when she was trying to address her complex needs as she battled breast cancer. Then, we shared Lisbet's story and our research about the power of Family Justice Centers in bringing all the services together under one roof for victims of child abuse, domestic violence, sexual assault, elder abuse, and human trafficking. The first Family Justice Center saw the power of collective hope early in its existence.

In the early years of the first Family Justice Center in the country—the San Diego Family Justice Center, with 25 agencies under one roof—Casey Gwinn and Gael Strack created a culture of professionals (cops, prosecutors, advocates, therapists, chaplains, and others) who believed they could save the lives of victims and stop violent offenders. Though no one was measuring hope in the staff and partners of the Center in those early years, they were clearly a group of high hope professionals with shared goals of saving lives and successfully prosecuting offenders. Homicides declined and convictions climbed. Collective hope and a culture of hope worked. Once they all believed they could do it, when survivors came to the Center for help, they felt it and believed it too. Survivors came in larger and larger numbers as they felt welcomed into a community with high hope professionals.

The San Diego Family Justice Center helped reduce the domestic violence homicide rate 90% in the City of San Diego. It was the power of collective hope among everyone that worked there that created a culture of hope. It worked in the San Diego Family Justice Center and it is now working in more than 100 Family Justice Centers across the country and around the world.

Victims are now flocking to Family Justice Centers and similar types of Centers because they make it easier for survivors to set goals and find pathways. Instead of having to navigate 10-15-20 agencies/places to get help—telling the story repeatedly—survivors can now come one place for everything they need.

Organizations that understand the science of hope and the challenges of trauma are providing the pathways and support to help survivors navigate more easily toward their goal of living safely and thriving after trauma. Easier access to help can influence the survivor's motivation as she or he navigates the pathways toward goal achievement.

If this support is provided in a coordinated way, the result is rising hope in the lives of those seeking help. Collective hope can also influence an entire community.

Community-wide hope

How does collective hope influence a community? In one study, we collected over 1,000 responses from a medium-sized urban city. While we discovered that individual hope was the most significant predictor of individual happiness among these community participants, collective hope was the most significant predictor of over-all community well-being. The same was found for individual and collective goal attainment. Individual hope is the most significant predictor of individual success but collective hope is the best predictor of a community's success. We were able to connect our survey responses to public health data for the community and found that both individual hope and collective hope were predictive of life expectancy. The higher Hope scores went for individuals and for the entire group, the longer people in the group lived. Finally, we found that collective hope was predictive of voter turnout (social action) for the mayoral election. If the whole community had rising hope, election turnout went up. These are exciting new findings for the power of hope not only for the individual but for considering a community's well-being.

Imagine if our civic leaders began to pay attention to the power of hope. How could a Chamber of Commerce use this information to advocate for economic development in recruiting new business? A hopeful community represents a tremendous resource for any leader. Imagine if every leader of a VA facility serving combat veterans focused on producing collective hope. How would struggling veterans benefit from a culture of hope?

How does collective hope influence the work place? We recently conducted studies to explore this idea. First, individual hope was found to be a significant buffer to burnout but collective hope was a better predictor of engagement in the workplace than individual hope. Collective hope was associated positively with job satisfaction and negatively with turnover. Employee turnover went down when hope went up. We also found that collective hope was stronger when employees believed that their supervisor cared for their well-being and valued their contribution to the team. We also found that ethical leadership behaviors were predictive of collective hope. The more honest the leaders, the greater the likelihood of collective hope.

We now want to take hope and implement it in the workplace just as others in the positive psychology movement have been advocating for in recent years. One concept that is foundational to our focus on a hope-centered workplace is called psychological capital.

Psychological Capital

University of Nebraska professor Fred Luthans, one of the leading thinkers in the positive psychology movement today, argues that employers should be shifting away from what is wrong with people and emphasizing what is right with people. He challenges employers to focus on strengths as opposed to weakness, resilience as opposed to vulnerability, and enhancing wellness as opposed to trying to remediate pathology. Luthans has articulated a concept known as psychological capital in focusing on how to improve employee performance and morale. Not surprisingly, hope is part of the equation. Luthans identifies four core components in what he calls psychological capital (PsyCap):

- **Self-efficacy**: having confidence to take on and put in the necessary effort to succeed at challenging tasks
- **Optimism**: making a positive attribution and expectation about succeeding now and in the future
- **Hope:** persevering toward goals and, when necessary, redirecting paths to goals in order to succeed
- **Resilience:** when beset by problems and adversity, sustaining and bouncing back and even beyond to attain success

Let's look briefly at each element.

Self-Efficacy—Self-efficacy, as we noted earlier, refers to the confidence you have about your ability to pursue and attain a specific goal. Confidence in your own abilities generally is a good thing and produces better outcomes than a low view of your abilities to pursue a goal or complete a task successfully.

Optimism—As we discussed earlier, optimism differs from hope. Optimism refers to the expectation that good outcomes will occur. While this future expectation is shared by both hope and optimism, hope includes both *pathways* thinking and the *willpower* to pursue selected pathways. Optimism is only the expectation itself.

Hope—Hope refers to an individual's motivation to succeed at a specific task in a set context and the way or means by which that task may be accomplished. The idea that we have discussed throughout the book is that you have *goals* you desire to achieve, you can identify *pathways* toward the goals, and you can direct and sustain your *willpower* toward the goal and pathways necessary to reach those goals = Hope rising.

Resilience—Resilience refers to the ability of an individual to bounce back from adversity, uncertainty, risk or failure, and adapt to changing and stressful life demands. One of our Camp HOPE America children, Jeanell, referred to it as a palm tree that bends all the way over in the wind but does not break. Truth.

Researchers have found that higher PsyCap (the combination of increases in these four key measurements for employees) leads directly to lower employee absenteeism, lower employee cynicism and intentions to quit, and higher job satisfaction, commitment, and organizational citizenship behaviors (discretionary behaviors that go beyond a job description to support and improve the organization).

Luthans has documented that there are significant relationships between the increased level of PsyCap and:

- desirable employee attitudes (job satisfaction, organizational commitment, psychological well-being),
- desirable employee behaviors (citizenship)
- multiple measures of performance (self, supervisor evaluations, and objective).
- undesirable employee attitudes (cynicism, turnover intentions, job stress, and anxiety)
- undesirable employee behaviors (deviance).

This is what a hope-centered workplace looks like. Employees have rising hope and a strong sense of mission that is far greater than simply having a job or working 8-5 and going home.

We need to teach to the test in the workplace. We need to focus on how to increase hope, self-efficacy, optimism, and resilience. It will change the way employees do their work. It will change our workplaces.

Here are some tips for encouraging PsyCap in your organization:

- **Self-efficacy:** Challenge employees to set clear, measurable and achievable goals;
- **Optimism:** Broadcast their success and the success of other employees;
- **Hope:** Give people a feeling of agency (the ability to make their own decisions) and help them to plan a way to succeed (pathways toward their goals);

- **Resilience:** Give people the resources, relationships and emotional support to help them recuperate from stress, vicarious trauma, conflict, failure, or changes in responsibility.

Perhaps most importantly, begin talking about hope and these core competencies that improve worker performance. We advocate for measuring ACEs (particularly in social services and mental health organizations) and hope in the place you work in on a regular basis. But measuring hope should be a non-negotiable. If you are not a supervisor, share this book with your supervisor and see if they are willing to consider it.

Vicarious Trauma and Self-Care

Perhaps the greatest enemy of individual hope in many workplaces is the impact of vicarious trauma. We touched on this earlier. Even if you have not experienced major personal trauma in your life, you can end up a person with low hope because of what others around have experienced and are relating to you. Vicarious trauma, referred to by some as compassion fatigue, is the impact of trauma on care providers or others that did not experience that trauma personally. Therapists, first responders, members of the clergy, and other helping professionals often experience vicarious trauma the most. There are primary victims in trauma such as violence or abuse, car accidents, or natural disasters and then there is secondary victimization, sometimes called secondary traumatic stress happening to those trying to help the primary victims.

We distinguish vicarious trauma from burnout. Burnout can come and go and people can mitigate it with a vacation or a change in jobs. Burnout is real and we will touch on it briefly later in this chapter. Vicarious trauma is much deeper. Vicarious trauma can produce stress, tension, anxiety, and even a preoccupation with the experiences of others that become difficult to get out of your mind. How a person responds to vicarious trauma can vary from individual to individual. For some, it might produce numbing where feelings get blocked or subdued. Others might end up in a persistent state of arousal like the hypervigilance we have seen in the direct victims of trauma. Vicarious trauma is usually most evident in sexual assault or domestic violence advocates or therapists who are hearing stories of great trauma every day and experiencing some of the impacts themselves even though they did not experience the underlying trauma being described.

Self-care is the antidote to vicarious trauma. Experts recommend different approaches but most of the approaches to self-care involve these key elements: Mindfulness; Community Support; Energy Discharge; and Focus on Wellbeing.

Mindfulness: As we have talked about multiple times in this book, breathing and movement that help us utilize sensory strategies often help. Bessel van der Kolk says 60 breaths with special focus on longer exhales than inhales will do powerful work in calming our bodies and minds. We do mindfulness with children at camp to help ground them at the beginning of each day and we do it at work at the beginning of staff meetings. Consciously slowing down your breathing and breathing deeply is part of the journey. Working to free your mind of stress-filled and consuming thoughts is part of the work of breathing exercises and mindfulness. Movement, including yoga, is the stretching and relaxing of your body that can help release stress and toxic energy trapped in your muscles and cells.

Community Support: Having good friends that you can share your feelings with after experiencing direct or indirect trauma is important. Pick friends that are empathic—that know how to show empathy and express care for you. They need to be friends that are not going to judge you or be shocked if you need to express dark and painful feelings.

Energy Discharge: Walking, going on an elliptical machine, or running is a great way to discharge energy. Strenuous physical movement is a healthy way to release energy from the body. Don't minimize the importance of sweating out some of your stress!

Focus on Wellbeing: Feed yourself well; Eat healthy; Sleep long enough to rejuvenate yourself; Avoid toxins whenever you can; and breathe deep often.

If you need professional support from a counselor or a therapist, do it. Don't view asking for some professional help as a weakness or a crutch. Sometimes we have both found it is hard to turn off what we do and we must creatively find ways to disconnect or get away from the stress and pain of our work. Vicarious trauma can impact your hope level. Left ignored and to its own devices, vicarious trauma will sap your energy for goal setting and your mental acumen for identifying pathways to your goals. Don't ignore it and don't pretend like you are a super hero. Everybody else knows you're not anyway so just admit it.

Burnout

Professional exhaustion and burnout differ from vicarious trauma but they too can play powerfully negative roles in damaging hope in our lives. Dr. Edy Greenblatt, a life coach and resiliency educator has identified the "Three Musketeers" for overcoming exhaustion and burnout:

- Gaining an understanding of what restores or depletes your energy (what energizes one person may deplete another);
- Challenging social tags such as "work" or "vacation" to identify your true restoration and depletion triggers;
- Becoming aware that, over time, your sources of depletion and restoration will change and you must therefore adapt.

These topics are great conversations to have with people in the workplace. There are also other ways to create work environments that are more conducive to rising hope.

Dr. George Everly at Johns Hopkins University argues for trying to create resilient organizational cultures for employees. He argues that people prosper from success so giving employees all the tools they need to succeed is a great foundation. But beyond that he advocates for formal and informal sub-groups in the workplace where they can build relationships with other employees. It sounds similar to the notion of Hope buddies we saw in the school research in Kansas. His main point: Encouragement, support, and mentoring are crucial. Interpersonal support at work is one of the strongest predictors of success. We would argue, based on the science of hope, that social support at work improves agency/motivation to set and pursue goals. Managing stress is also crucial. This means employers and workplaces should be teaching self-care techniques and even hosting activities that model good stress management and balanced living. If every wellness program measured hope and taught to the test (including a focus on physical fitness, nutrition, and stress management), companies would be stunned at the increase in wellness and decrease in absenteeism among their employees.

Most recently, Rich Fernandez, who has done work on learning and organizational development at Google and eBay has recommend five strategies for a hope-centered workplace:

- Practice mindfulness to manage and minimize your stress
- Compartmentalize your work (keeping it separate from other parts of your life) to enhance your productivity and decrease cognitive strain
- Take "breaks" where you "detach" to replenish your natural mental focus, clarity, and energy cycles

- Develop mental agility to respond thoughtfully and constructively to stress
- Cultivate compassion for yourself (be kind to yourself) and for others to enhance your well-being

Five Recommendations to Have High Hope at Work

Shane Lopez provided five recommendations out of his research about workers with high hope. They should go on our mirrors along with high worth statements about who we are and can be.

- *Test Drive the Future*—This connects to the ability to imagine what your perfect job looks like and then you can start setting goals to create it. Think through what you are aiming for and whether you can create it at your current job or need to pursue it somewhere else.
- Some of the most successful companies with the happiest employees are now implementing "Dream Time" for 30 minutes each week where every employee is challenged to commit to their dream or dreams in public, then consult weekly with a designated "dream manager" on the staff of the organization, and then spend 30 minutes on Friday mornings pursuing their dreams. The dreams don't have to be work-related but they do have to agree to pursue them. This is a great way to boost engagement, productivity, and well-being at work.
- *Trust Your Gut*—When you are interviewing for a job, don't just talk to those on interview panels. Ask to talk to other potential co-workers. Ask if they feel supported in the workplace and by those they work with. If you are already in the workplace, hang out with people that make you feel good and stay away from those that pull you down. Your gut will give you a strong sense of this before and after you are working for a company.
- *Play to Your Strengths*—This connects to our discussion about strength-based approaches above but comes from your own perspective. What are you good at? Can you focus your job on what you are good at? If you can't, you probably need another job. But if you can spend most of your time doing what you do best, you will be happier at work.
- *Craft Your Job*—This is related to playing to your strengths but really focuses more on organizing your day to give you the most motivation. Is it best for you to do your least favorite work in the morning, and then do what you love the most in the afternoon? Or will you do better later in the day if you have truly enjoyed your work in the morning? It also relates to "spend and send."

Spend time with those you enjoy at work and those who care about you the most. *Send* emails to those you don't really care about and those who suck the life right out of you. Take control of crafting your job because the research is clear: Happiness and hope at work depend on loving your job and jobs you love are made, not found.

- *Shop for the Right Boss*—If you are a boss, be that hope-centered leader we have talked about. If you are not the boss, find the right one if you can. Find a way to report to someone that inspires you, encourages you, and gives you hope.

What would your employer find if they measured hope in your workplace? What could change in your workplace if your employer measured it? We need hope-centered workplaces in this country. If you are the boss, what can you do to implement the science of hope in your company or organization? If you are not the boss, who needs a copy of this book for their birthday?! We need to set our goals higher in the workplace than avoiding sexual harassment and abuse of employees. Let's aim for rising hope.

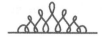

Chapter 21

The End of Shame

"Shame derives its power from being unspeakable."
—Brené Brown

Anna O.

In the late 19th century, a French neurologist named Jean-Martin Charcoat first identified the relationship between childhood sexual abuse and profound symptoms later in adulthood during his study of "hysteria" in women. "Hysteria" was the diagnosis for women with major mental health issues that ended up in a hospital (asylum) outside of Paris. It was considered a female disorder and was grounded in profound cultural bias against women and girls. Charcoat was a well-known French doctor that began studying the phenomenon of "hysteria" first. He soon discovered that the deeply troubled women in the asylum, once interviewed or hypnotized and then interviewed, disclosed consistent stories of victimization during childhood by rape, incest, and other forms of sexual abuse. The disclosure of their stories was a collaborative effort between the doctors and the patients. Early on it became clear that if patients could tell their stories, they would begin to heal.

Charcoat's work attracted the interest of Sigmund Freud, today known as the father of modern psychology. Sigmund Freud traveled to Paris to study Charcoat's work and then began focusing on documenting the stories of women diagnosed with hysteria in Vienna as well. Freud called the process of helping them remember and telling their stories as "catharsis" and later "psycho-analysis." Joseph Breuer, a colleague of Freud in Vienna, joined his research effort. Breuer has a patient known as "Anna O." Anna O. dubbed the process of figuring out what happened to the women as little girls and then helping them talk about it as "the talking cure." Freud and Breuer found, just as Charcoat had found in France, that the more they talked about what had happened to them the faster their recovery seemed to take place.

Sigmund Freud became deeply focused on the relationship between "hysteria" and childhood sexual abuse and authored a major piece on the topic in 1896. He wrote in part: "...at the bottom of every case of hysteria there are one or more premature sexual experiences, occurrences which belong to the earliest years of childhood..." Dr. Judith Herman tells the story best of what happened after Freud issued his Aetiology of Hysteria: "Hysteria was so common among women that if his patients' stories were true, and if his theory was correct, he would be forced to conclude that what he called 'perverted acts against children' were endemic, not only among the proletariat of Paris, where he had first studied hysteria, but also among the respectable bourgeois families of Vienna, where he had established his practice. This idea was simply unacceptable. It was beyond credibility." What did Freud do? He recanted his findings, covered up his research, and never again spoke publicly about his earlier findings. He depended on the wealthy families of Vienna for his living. Surely, he could not accuse them of participating in endemic child sexual abuse."

Freud's cowardice about confronting child sexual abuse in Europe in the late 18th Century helped pull a shroud of shame over millions of victims of trauma and abuse that would come after the "hysteria" patients of the Freud's day. Freud could no longer even listen to their stories and give them any credibility. He moved away from the notion of "catharsis" and chose "psychoanalysis" and launched the dominant psychological theory of the 20th Century—grounded in a denial of the reality of women experiencing abuse. For Freud, sexuality became the central focus of the inquiry. But it was not focused on sexually abusive conduct, it was focused on obsession with sex by women and men. Psychoanalysis became the study of people's fantasies and unquenchable sexual desire, dissociated from the reality of the experience for women and girls. By the beginning of the 1900s, with no evidence that the victims of sexual abuse were lying, Freud decided that the very volume of such complaints must prove them to be false.

Judith Hermann identified Freud's dishonesty in her seminal book *Trauma and Recovery* in 1992. After Freud's cowardice, it took 90 years for Dr. Vincent Felitti and the ACE Study to re-discover the truth and provide the clinical documentation that corroborated the long-term impacts of child physical and sexual abuse. If our goal is rising hope, we can never ignore or shame victims again. We must never sacrifice truth on the altar of expediency. Freud sacrificed the truth to save his career, protect his livelihood, and avoid the reality of a culture that subjugated, demeaned, abused, and minimized women and girls. We still fight those battles today but we must win them if are going to see rising hope in the lives of women, men, and children in this country. Shame derives its power from being unspeakable. Sigmund Freud, the father of modern psychology, imposed a gag order on sexually abused girls and women and gave shame greater power.

Shame is that intensely painful feeling or experience of believing that we are flawed, broken, and unworthy. Sometimes it comes from something we have done or failed to do but it also often comes from things others have done to us.

It is hard not to reflect today on how Freud's decisions haunt so many with shame today. The #metoo campaign continues to provide a platform for millions of women (and men) to share their stories of sexual harassment, abuse, and molestation. Stories they have been ashamed or embarrassed to share for many years. We both shared their own experiences of being molested as children. Why didn't we talk about it before now? Shame. Embarrassment. Self-blame. We must declare again that shame is an enemy of hope. But the reluctance to be vulnerable and tell the truth about our lives and what has happened to us is understandable just as Freud's decision to ignore the truth was understandable.

Even today, some are fighting back against millions of women coming forward to share their stories of abuse and arguing that if there really were that many men harassing and abusing women that would mean it is almost an epidemic! And if all these powerful women that are sharing their stories are telling the truth—writers, politicians, actresses, and business leaders—then that would mean there are men in the highest levels of government, business, the media, and the faith community that are abusing women. Could it really be true? Could there be that much abuse hidden in the culture?

Even the reporting is wading into it carefully—calling it "harassment," "inappropriate sexual behavior in the workplace," and "sexual misconduct." But the truth must be told and we must call it what it is. Freud first called it "perverted acts." But as he began to back away from his conclusions, he referred to it as "premature sexual experiences." As the stories continue to break, if we are going to lift the shame from victimization in this country—we need to call men who sexually assault women what they are: Rapists.

We also need to recognize that Anna O. had it right. Empowering victims of abuse to tell their story is cathartic—it is the "talking cure"—true for adults and for children.

We love the research being done that is finding that the talking cure works for children. And the sooner the better after the trauma. The Yale Child Study Center in New Haven, Connecticut has developed a short, five-week program called Child and Family Traumatic Stress Intervention (CFTSI) that is showing that helping a child talk about an experience like child abuse or witnessing domestic violence and giving them tools to process it has great healing power. CFTSI also engages the child's care provider as well to give them both the ability to talk about trauma, understand what kinds of reactions they might experience (normal reactions to an abnormal experience), and then some tools to learn how to reduce or avoid a toxic stress response can help the child overcome the trauma more quickly. This opens the door for both a parent and child to see themselves as a "team" to help reduce the impacts of the trauma. It also opens the door to new goal setting and pathways thinking for the child, and rising hope.

"The Talking Cure" Led to a Woman with High Hope

Once we make the trauma-informed shift from what is wrong with you, to what happened to you, we can begin the healing and move toward a pathway to hope. Though virtually all doctors investigating "hysteria" and its connection to "childhood sexual abuse," including Freud, recanted their work and ignored the truth of their findings, Anna O. never recanted her story. Anna O. found her way forward though being abandoned by Freud and Joseph Breuer. She recovered from her post-traumatic stress and went on to become a pioneer in the early women's liberation movement including working as a social worker helping other women. Her real name was Bertha Pappenheim. During her amazing life, Bertha founded a feminist organization for Jewish women, ran an orphanage for girls, and campaigned against the sexual exploitation of women and children. Philosopher Martin Buber wrote these words shortly after her death: "I not only admired her but loved her, and will love her until the day I die. There are people of spirit and there are people of passion, both less common than one might think. Rarer still are the people of passion and spirit. But rarest of all is a passionate spirit. Bertha Pappenheim was a woman with just such a spirit. Pass on her memory. Be witnesses that it still exists."

In her will, Bertha Pappenheim made clear what she wanted if people visited her grave. She asked that each visitor leave a small stone "as a quiet promise…to serve the mission of women's duties and women's joy…unflinchingly and courageously." It is on our bucket lists now—leaving a small stone at Bertha's grave.

We have both told our full stories of childhood trauma in this book. An end to shame. Courageous men, women, and teens have shared their stories throughout this book. An end to shame. The result: Hope rising. It is the power of collective hope as we all share our truth here. The power of the talking cure. Jesus said it another way, "The truth will set you free." It will set you free to start setting goals and looking for pathways to achieve those goals with others cheering you on and standing with you on the way. There are many women today in America talking in the #metoo campaign that are finally feeling the freedom of telling the truth and being believed about what they have endured. An end to shame.

The Path Out of Shame Runs Through Vulnerability

Brené Brown talks about vulnerability as the pathway out of shame and toward connection to others. Brené Brown calls shame the "master emotion." Shame is our fear that we don't measure up, that we can never measure up because of what we have done or what has been done to us. Shame will eat at you like a cancer. But we can deal with it. We can find people that will come along side us and offer us grace, encouragement and affirmation. We can tell the truth to those that love us. We can find honest people that will view our vulnerability as courage. And the loving acceptance of others will help us let go of our shame and open the door to self-esteem. Brown says it so well, "Empathy is the antidote to shame." We need to offer empathy and find those who will offer it to us. It will help us become people who realize we are gifted, talented, creative, and capable.

Those with low hope in our research seem to be people who are terrified to be truly seen and known. Those with low hope let fear rule their lives. It is often connected to trauma or fear of not measuring up, but fear or anxiety become their closest friend.

The sooner we can model and teach children about authenticity, honesty, forgiveness, and empathy the better. It is all part of the soil we must cultivate to grow rising hope and mitigate the power of adversity that will otherwise send children toward rage, narcissism, and an endless struggle to put down others to lift themselves up.

We would have less predators in this world if we taught rage-filled children how to navigate through their rage—moving higher on the Hope Continuum. We would have less narcissists if we could help trauma-exposed children understand that they can be extraordinary without putting down others or elevating themselves. If we start younger with helping children and teens find purpose in their lives, it would matter. It is hard to be a narcissist when you learn young that hope is believing in yourself, believing in others, and believing in your dreams. Children with high Hope scores don't spend their time trying to get attention, causing drama, throwing fits, blaming others, or taking credit for things they did not do. Adults with high Hope scores don't spend their time playing the martyr, manipulating others, or triangulating.

The greatest battle most of us will ever fight is the temptation to run from honest relationships and hide ourselves in achievement, (false) superiority, or past victimization. We said it early in the book. Fear is our opportunity for courage. Courage at the end of the day is always a choice. The choice to share our story and embrace our weaknesses and inadequacies is the beginning of vulnerability. Choosing courage, telling our truth, being vulnerable gives us the opportunity to experience rising hope in our lives.

Forgive Yourself

During our journey through and out of trauma and adversity, we often struggle with guilt. This is particularly true if we made mistakes or decisions that played a role in the trauma or adversity we experienced. During a conference on Sexual Assault Response Best Practices in New Orleans several years ago, Casey shared with the audience some of his personal struggles because of trauma in his past and some bad decisions he felt he had made. A therapist named Jill came up to him and said, "Casey, I give you permission to forgive yourself. You need to forgive yourself, let it go, and claim freedom from it." Casey doesn't know if it was her body language, the way she took both his hands in hers, or just the caring look on her face, but he immediately realized just how much self-blame and shame he was carrying about a variety of things. Replaying his own mistakes over and over. Casey promised her he would spend time alone and with his God and work on her challenge. It might be a message many of us need. Sometimes our biggest issue is not someone else forgiving us, it is our own willingness and choice to forgive ourselves. Do you need to forgive yourself for anything? Do you need to let something go so you can start better positive self-talk?

We have both put a saying up on our mirrors during the writing of this book.

"I am important, deserving, loving, intelligent, worthy, compassionate, beautiful, creative, inspiring, brave, true, strong, and able. I will keep acknowledging it until I finally realize it for myself."

We should all post it. We all need it.

Give the Gift of Hope Instead of Shame

Nina

Nina has worked as a hair dresser for more than 20 years. She was a nurse before she started doing hair. She has strong empathy and transference—she feels the pain of others and loves to encourage those who have suffered tough times. She knows that pain. Her dad left right after her birth and she never saw him again.

We interviewed Nina for the book after randomly meeting her at a New Year's Day party. As we explained the science of hope to her, she was intrigued. "Everyone has so much pain they hold in and they often tell me their story while I am doing their hair," she said. "They have learned that hair dressers and stylists are not the kind of people that are going to shame them or judge them." She said she has heard every story imaginable about pain, loss, and trauma. "One of my clients just went through the death of her 22-year-old son. It has been so devastating." We asked her how she tries to support them and encourage them. She said, "First, I am a great listener and I know how to ask good questions."

After she learned about the science around hope, she said she could easily ask her clients about small or large goals in their life. She loved the idea of then getting them to think about the steps they would need to take to achieve their goals. "It would be a simple addition to what I already do with all of my clients."

We loved to see Nina thinking about how she could do a few simple things to increase hope and mitigate shame. Shame always looks back. Hope always looks forward. Nina is a hope giver and helping her clients to look forward more will produce rising hope.

Agustin

We saw earlier in the book that some of the most rage-filled, low hope men on the planet are stranglers of women. Most victims don't call it strangulation. They call it "choking." But applying pressure to the neck of another person that cuts off air flow or blood flow in the arteries or veins is actually strangulation. One of the most popular training programs of Alliance for HOPE International is a four-day program where communities bring multi-disciplinary teams (police officer, prosecutor, advocate, and medical professional) to learn how to handle non-fatal strangulation cases. We talked earlier about this program. It is called the Training Institute on Strangulation Prevention (www.strangulationtraininginstitute.com).

Agustin was a detective from Maine who came to one of the four day courses with a multi-disciplinary team last year. Gael Strack, the founder of the Institute, has added a session on the science of hope that Casey now teaches for all the attendees of the course. After Agustin heard about the power of hope he started to think about how he could change the way he did his job to increase hope in the lives of survivors in the strangulation cases he investigates. At the end of the course, when participants were asked how they would do their job differently when they got home, Agustin raised his hand. "I need to be a better hopegiver when I do my job. Now that I understand how to increase hope, I am going to start asking each survivor some different questions at the end of every interview."

Casey and Gael were intrigued. Casey asked him what he was going to ask. He said, "After I get all the evidence, I am going to tell her it is not her fault to reduce the shame. I am going to tell her how proud I am of the way she has stayed alive with such a dangerous man in her life. Then, I am going to ask her to name one goal she has in her life looking forward." It would be an opportunity for a future-orientation for someone thinking about terrible pain in her past. "Then, I am going to ask her to think about the first step she needs to take to move toward her goal," Agustin said.

Casey asked him what he thought it would do for the victim. Agustin did not hesitate. "She has just suffered the worst trauma of her life. She probably thought she was going to die while he was choking her and she had no power over what was happening. It sucked the hope right out of her life. By helping her think about a goal and a pathway, I will be helping her increase hope again, just a little bit, in her life."

Alliance for HOPE International has a national partnership with Paul Mitchell Schools to re-use the old doll heads that hairdressers practice on during their two years of training. Winn Claybaugh, the co-founder of Paul Mitchell Schools, got excited about the opportunity to ask his hair dressers to donate the used doll heads to detectives like Agustin so that victims can demonstrate on doll heads how they were strangled. Detectives can then take pictures and no one has to place their hands again on a victim's neck to get demonstrative evidence of the assault to show to a judge or jury how the perpetrator applied pressure to her neck. We love the synergy of hairdressers and detectives working together to reduce shame and increase hope.

Our goal is for every professional in every type of job to begin thinking about how they can help reduce shame and increase hope in others by the way they do their jobs. It is all about helping people think about goals, motivation to pursue their goals, and the pathways they need to take to see their goals become a reality.

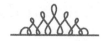

Chapter 22

Hope Rising: Leaving a Legacy of Hope

"Carve your name on hearts, not on tombstones."
—Shannon L. Alder

The Stories of Hope
We have told the stories about the science of hope in this book. They are not all happy endings. And hope is not always linear. They are real people though. Think back to the beginning. Lance on the run with Maddie in pursuit. Diane and Joe at Sharp Hospital. David. Ellen. Dana. Inocente. Rick. Darcy, Larry, Shawna, and Matt. Nora. Jardon. Dalia. Allan. Colette. Laura. Chris. Katie. Devon. Stephen. Justin. Byron. Bill. Emeka. Jerome. Dan. Barbara. Gemma. Lisbet. Emerson. Lila. Tricia. Karianne. Mike. Carrie. John. Michael. Yusra. Maya. Jim. Casey. Chan. Harvey. Anna. Nina. Agustin.

Rising hope is, at its core, about the choices people make and the relationships they form. Whether you are a person of faith or not, what outlives you will be your investment in the lives of children, family, and friends who will live their lives differently because of you. We believe in life after death and we believe that decisions and actions in this life matter in the context of eternity, but the truth is that your legacy in this life will be lived out by those that remain after you are gone. We have all made mistakes and we have all lived at times with low hope. Some of us live with the guilt of negatively impacting hope in other people's lives. But there is good news. If you have breath, it is not too late. You can set different goals and pursue different pathways.

Where do you start? Do you need to clear the decks with anyone that your actions have hurt? Forgive yourself first. Then, reach out to your friends, family members, children or grandchildren if forgiveness is necessary with others. Then, start thinking about what will help you most to raise your own Hope score and think about others you know that need rising hope in their lives. It is not too late to create a legacy of hope from your life.

Legacy discussions are difficult. We cannot decide personally what our legacy will be. Others will decide that for us after we are gone. Thinking about legacy means thinking about the finite nature of life. Nobody makes it out of this life alive. We all have a beginning and an end. Casey began life in 1960. Chan began life in 1965. Right now, we are in the -. Our life is the dash. There will be another year put after the dash. It might be 2018. It might be 2025 or 2035. We don't know. We don't get to decide the first number or the last number. But we do get to decide what the dash means in between the two numbers. And the dash is always good things and bad things. No one does all "good" and no one does all "bad." We can choose to live with the shame and guilt of our mistakes or we can focus on the opportunities we have to do good things for those we love and those God brings into our lives before the second number gets tagged onto our dash.

We all need to surround ourselves with people that encourage and affirm us. Negative, critical people are like a cancer. But people who speak grace and forgiveness and become vulnerable with us so we can know that we are not alone—those are the people we need to be around.

No one with an empty emotional gas tank can do much to offer hope and encouragement to others around him or her. Burned out, hopeless people don't have much to offer. Chan administered the Adult Hope Scale to homeless service providers in Tulsa, Oklahoma a few years ago. They were stunned to find out that their Hope scores were barely above the scores of the homeless population they were serving every day. It was a wake call for policy makers as well. They needed to focus on increasing hope in the lives of the service providers if they are going to increase hope in the people on the streets of Tulsa.

You cannot give what you do not have. If you do not have hope, you cannot give hope. This makes it crucial that you start keeping track of yours. Go to <u>www.</u>

hopescore.org and take your Hope score if you have not already. Benchmark it and track it as you go forward in life. Maybe you need to create an account for each of your family members as well and have them take it. You will see that we also want you to take the ACE Index. If your ACE score is zero, you should be thankful. For most reading this book, you will have an ACE score greater than zero. No shame. And you don't have to tell others if you are not ready. But it is best to know your ACE score before you can see the power of your rising Hope score. And don't forget about vicarious trauma even if you have not experienced much trauma yourself. If you are in the helping, first responder, and serving professions, you still need to take care of yourself. The impact of vicarious trauma (the trauma others are experiencing being shared with you) is significant and cumulative. You end up needing the same kinds of care and support that those you are helping need. You need to be loved and encouraged. You need to maintain and build up your own Hope score so that you can benefit from the increased resiliency that comes along with it.

Learn to Love Yourself

Jesus talked about the importance of loving your neighbor as yourself. Did you catch the key piece of that? You need to make sure you love yourself in order to be able to love others. And if you don't find that you love yourself, you need to take the steps to find your way back to that place of loving yourself, valuing who you are, and who you are becoming. It might take some counseling and professional help. It did for both of us. It might take the courage to be really honest with those around you who can love and support you. Brené Brown has some great quotes in her book, *Daring Greatly*. One is: "*Courage starts with showing up and letting ourselves be seen.*" Another is: "*Vulnerability sounds like truth and feels like courage. Truth and courage aren't always comfortable, but they're never weakness.*" Our journey in writing this book has been a difficult one, but a freeing one. We have shared more of our personal stories than we were planning. But the deeper we looked at our own research, the more obvious the need to be transparent became for both of us. Being honest about the past helps us start looking forward. And hope is all about the ability to look forward to who we are becoming and what we can be and do.

Two years ago, Casey interviewed each of his adult children while writing *Cheering for the Children*. It was a daunting exercise that led to deep and honest conversation with each of them. We think it provides some great insight into this book. Here are the questions he asked:

How would you describe growing up in our home in general terms?
Do you feel we expressed our love for you enough?
Gary Chapman says there are five love languages:

- *Words of Affirmation*
- *Acts of Service*
- *Receiving Gifts*
- *Quality Time*
- *Physical Touch*

How would you rank those five concepts in how you best experience love and support?

How did we do in meeting those needs based on the way you best experience feeling loved?

What are your best memories?

What are your most difficult memories?

What do you think I did best as a parent?

What do you think Mom did best as a parent?

What things did I do as a Dad that caused you pain or difficulty in life?

Are there things you saw in Mom or me as a parent that you want to do differently when you become a parent?

Do you think we encouraged you enough? Were there times when you needed more encouragement or support and we did not provide it?

How could we have encouraged or affirmed you more?

Are there other things you wish we had done or things you wish we had not done with you or said to you?

The interviews led to interesting conversations about goals, motivation, and pathways in their lives that traced back to things that happened in childhood—both good and bad. Some powerful things jumped out from interviews with each of his children—things he never realized the power of until they shared it with him in retrospect:

- Individual trips and special activities with each child separately
- Storytelling where they made up stories together
- Family vacations where the family was all together and there were few distractions (camping and houseboating with no electronics)

- Notes, cards, and letters written to them expressing love, affirmation, and personalized encouragement, picturing their special future (especially when it was not for a birthday or formal occasion)
- Affection and physical touch throughout their growing up years
- Regular, verbalized "I love yous" and clear statements of appreciation for who they were or about character traits he and Beth saw in them
- Being there for their events, activities, sports teams, and significant moments
- Asking questions about their days, lives, and relationships
- Praying with them every night and debriefing their day (especially when they were younger)
- Creating a home where all their friends wanted to come and hang out
- Messaging his daughters about high standards for boys in their lives (don't settle)
- Teaching his son how to respect and honor girls and women by how he treated his mother
- His daughters seeing how he treated their mother which helped them know what kind of man they wanted in their lives
- Helping each child set goals and think about ways to accomplish those big or small goals they were setting in their lives.

We both wish we had done these interviews when we were raising our children. We both think mid-course corrections would have been best. We didn't have Hope scores when we raised our kids but we are thankful we can propose using them when our grandchildren are old enough.

Lessons Learned from Two Old Guys

As we wrap up this book, let us share a few of the lessons we have learned from the research for this book. We have put together some reflections on leaving a legacy of hope in the lives of children and those we love. Most of this book has been written to adults. But as we reflect on creating legacies of hope, we want to focus on children and teens and how we can help them find rising hope.

We all leave a legacy to our own children and other children in our lives. If your experience with your father and mother was healthy and positive, you have an advantage in leaving a healthy legacy to your children. If your experience had negative elements as most of us did, your goal should be to leave a different or better legacy for your children and the children that come into your life.

1. **Teach your children (and friends) to be hope-centered**—Learn to use the language of hope in everything you do and then teach those you love and others around you in the workplace and other interactions. Once they understand the language of hope and the research, you will all talk and think differently about your lives, your goals, and your futures;

2. **When the time is right, make it OK to talk about the bad stuff of life**—We measure ACE scores in 11 year olds, older teens, and adults. We think that it is OK to start talking in age appropriate terms with children about things that make them mad, sad, or scared. We need to create honest communication with children if we are ever going to expect them to be honest, vulnerable adults;

3. **You can never be too positive or affirming with children**—Find ways every day to encourage children and praise them for character you see in them, effort made in various tasks and responsibilities, and ways they encourage or help others. When children tend toward negative statements in their own lives such as "I will never be good at science", help them think about re-framing toward a hopeful statement like "Science is not my best subject, but there are things I can do to improve my understanding and work";

4. **Ask questions that expect narrative answers**—Too often as we dialogue with children we ask them "How was your day at school?" "Fine"—End of conversation. We have found that asking them about their favorite part of the day and asking them about their toughest part of the day produced more discussion than one-word answers or "Yes" or "No" questions;

5. **Empathy always opens doors**—It is generally always better to find a way to connect with children and let them know that their experience is similar to yours in some way. Therapist David Wexler calls it "twinship" experiences. If children don't think you can relate and you don't help validate their feelings or experiences, it is tough to make a connection that can grow into a hope giving relationship;

6. **Listen more than you talk**—As men, we tend to want to be fixers. We want to fix things. Tell us your problem and we will help you solve it. But children, especially trauma-exposed children, need to tell you what happened. They need you to ask good questions. They need to validate and not judge them. They don't need you to try to fix it or push past their feelings quickly. Throughout the book, from the ACE study on, we have seen the power of listening and kind, thoughtful responsiveness;

7. **Run from negative people**—Many studies have found that negativity is not good for your health. Negative attitudes increase chronic stress and anxiety, upset the body's hormone balance, deplete brain chemicals required for happiness, and compromise the immune system. Negativity is often connected to toxic emotions such as guilt, shame, rage, self-loathing, regret, bitterness, and resentment.

Negative children will suck the hope right out of positive children. Children and adults know who the negative people are, but seldom run from them. They are the naysayers, the devil's advocates, and the critics who try to cast doubt on our abilities, the viability of our goals, and sometimes even our integrity in the struggle. We must all heed one message: Run!

The people that fit into this category say things like: "You have to be rich to do something like that." "No one in our family has ever amounted to anything." "Don't try to act like you are better than we are." "That's crazy talk." "Aren't you a little too old for fantasies like that?" "What makes you so special?" "Don't make the rest of us look bad."

In fact, children need to know that the bigger their goals and dreams, the more likely they are to attract critics and naysayers. Sometimes they are voices from the past. "You have always been a failure." "Do you remember when you tried to…? You failed then just like you will fail now." "What makes you think you can do that when you couldn't even…?" The truth is that statements like that are more about the low hope in the life of the speaker than they are about you. Those with low hope are the naysayers and negative ones that will show up when you try to focus on increasing hope in your life. Low hope people say things like, "Whatever happens, happens." "It is what it is." "There's nothing I can do about it anyway." Coming from others, call it what it is—messages attacking hope. Those messages must be processed and then repelled like a toxin we need to wash off our skin quickly.

It gets harder if those negative messages are coming from those we care about—from a spouse or dear friend. But the bottom line is that negative messaging neutralizes hope. You must find cheerleaders and supporters that will cheer you on, encourage you, and believe in you. Teach your children and grandchildren to do the same thing—run from negative people and surround themselves with positive people;

8. **Surround yourself with positive role models**—Let's change the last recommendation, a negative goal into a positive goal. Teach children to surround themselves with positive friends and mentors. High hope friends

will help you and the children in your life think about higher hope. Just like the Lawrence, Kansas school research we discussed, teach your children to pick good Hope buddies;

9. **Try to be trauma-informed in your responses**—We have looked at how trauma impacts human beings. We have seen how children act out because of trauma and often engage in behaviors that we don't like and want to discourage. But if we get distracted by their behavior and focus on it, we will not help them process the underlying trauma that is causing the behavior;

   For all the complex work being done by professionals around "trauma-informed care" and "trauma-informed practices," we remain convinced that being trauma-informed means we are compassionate, kind, and loving in our response to what children (and adults) have gone through. We don't blame or shame children or adults if we are sensitive to the trauma they have experienced. We listen and let them share their pain and loss instead of trying to steer them to only talk about the things we want to talk about in their story. We try to help them see that they are not abnormal or suffering from a "disorder" because of the way they reacted to a very abnormal situation. Then, we can begin to help them focus on hope. Survivors of trauma need trauma-informed and hope-centered people around them;

10. **Focus on strengths not on weaknesses or deficits**—We should always look at the strengths that children evidence amidst the pain or the trauma they are experiencing. The strengths they have will allow them to move forward. Focusing on their failures or their weaknesses will not help them overcome them. Rising hope will reduce the impact of their weaknesses. Focusing on their weaknesses will only drag them down;

11. **Engage in healthy physical affection**—Children, especially abused children, need to know what healthy, non-sexual affection feels like. They need to see and feel the universal language of affection—soft touches, hugs, gentle touches of the head and hair, hand holding when appropriate, and even kisses on the forehead or cheek. When Chan's teacher/coach put his arm around Chan's shoulder on a basketball court, that was life-changing, healthy physical affection. This is always a controversial subject in a world filled with abuse of children. But children need love and affection and we all need to figure out how to express affection in a way that is appropriate, done with permission, and non-threatening. We all need affection in our lives and children who have experienced trauma and abuse probably need it more than other children. Most children get it naturally but when physical touch has

been experienced as sexual or physical abuse we must not then refrain from any touch or affection with those children. They need it more than ever;

12. **Use your power and influence to bless children**—Adults have enormous power and influence in the lives of children. Most of the children who have experienced violence and abuse have suffered at the hands and words of adults who have misused their power and influence. Caring, loving adults must counteract that misuse of power with positive use of our position. Children long for approval and are shaped by the modeling that adults provide to them. Even teenagers who often describe their parents as idiots and morons still say that approval or disapproval of their parents is one of the most significant social forces in their lives. We need to use this power to build them up and help them feel blessed and favored;

13. **Say you are sorry when you need to**—It is healthy and good for parents to apologize. Sadly, it is way too rare. Our children have all said they wished we had apologized more when we did something wrong or reacted inappropriately. All of us should apologize more but not flippantly. Save it for when you really screw up and everyone knows it. You are not fooling anybody by pretending you were right when a child that your mistake impacted knows just how wrong you were. Humility and transparency opens the door to better relationships that puts you in a better place to encourage your children to pursue their goals and dreams;

14. **Become an expert on each child and an expert in the science of hope**—Whether your own children or the children of others, you need to become an expert in the uniqueness of each child. Children, even in the same family, are so totally different. Learn to study children, see their personality traits, see how they deal with different situations and understand their strengths and weaknesses. Don't try to fit them into a box or into the image of the child you think they are or want them to be. Some children are more naturally optimistic. Some children naturally gravitate toward higher hope. Study every child. Figure it out. Do they need a focus on agency in their *goals*? Do you remember the elements of *willpower* from the Children's Hope Scale? A child's subjective assessment of their own coping abilities in life—A child's perception of how they are doing in relation to other kids—A child's sense of how things in their past can help them in the future. Maybe you need focus on those areas. Or do they need a focus on pathways in their lives. Do you remember the *waypower* elements? A child's ability to get things in life that are important to them—A child's ability to think up ways to solve

problems—A child's determination to find ways to solve a problem even if other kids want to give up. Maybe this is where you need to focus your conversations. Trust the research. If you can improve their Hope scores based on how they rate themselves on each of these statements, children will do better in life in almost every arena;

15. **Help children re-goal when they need to adjust**—Re-goaling is where hope meets courage. When a child has a goal, but it becomes clear that there is no pathway or the child realizes that the goal does not matter as much as he or she thought at another time, a child can adjust the goal. It might take a slight adjustment. It might mean they pick a totally different goal. It is better to change a goal when there is no pathway than to descend into frustration, anger, rage, despair, or apathy by sticking with a goal that is not viable.

Final Reflections

We know the negative impacts of trauma and adversity in all of our lives. We know the enormous costs of trying to deal with the consequences of unmitigated trauma and toxic stress in the lives of children and adults in the health care system. We know the legacy of violence and abuse and the impacts they cause in the lives of children and later in their lives as adults. We know we can lose our ability to hope well. But we also know rising hope can change everything. The questions are now before us: Are we willing to invest the time and the resources to change the probabilities for those with high ACE scores and low levels of hope? Are we willing to help adults leave a different legacy for their children through their own rising Hope scores? Are we willing to commit our lives to pursuing goals, motivation, and pathways and surround ourselves with people that want to do the same?

It is Time to Act

Each of us can do something. First, we must ensure that we are high Hope score people. Second, we need to keep our scores high by working at it consistently. Third, we need to decide how to help others—adults and children to find their way to higher hope. We need our families to be cultures of hope. We need our marriages to be cultures of hope. Some have the power and influence to change public policy in America. Some can get an employer to start focusing on hope in the workplace. Others can focus on restoring hope to combat veterans across the country. Others have the power to invest far more corporate and philanthropic dollars in organizations that are raising Hope scores in at-risk and high-risk children and teens. Others can raise awareness about the science of hope in one school, church, business, or community organization.

We can all invest our time and resources in supporting organizations doing trauma-informed, hope-centered work to change the endings for children and adults struggling with low hope. On a personal level, everyone can decide to encourage and affirm their own children and grandchildren more actively. What will your legacy be? What will you do to help the children in your life have a different legacy than their parents or stepparents? We each have choices to make every day in how we can express love for the children of this generation and the next generation. Our choices today will impact eternity through the lives of those we love. It is our prayer that we will all leave a legacy of rising hope everywhere.

When…

When we feel trapped in the pain of today, hope reminds us we need not be there forever

When we feel stuck in looking back, hope calls to us to look forward

When we have given everything to others, hope helps us replenish our heart, mind, and body

When we are demoralized, hope can point us toward friends to lift our spirits

When we lose our way, hope can give us back a roadmap for our lives

When we fear the worst, hope reminds us that God is still in control

When we are hurting from the actions of others, hope is a pathway to resilience

When we must accept the consequences of our mistakes, hope lifts us out of the shame

When our heart is broken, hope offers us to the courage to look forward to healing

When the diagnosis is grim, hope calls us to the battle for survival

When we are forced to sit back and wait on a dream, hope gives us the patience to trust

When we feel bound in the darkness of despair, hope reminds us that there is a way to the light

When a dream does not come true, hope lights the fire to dream again

When we feel rejected and abandoned, hope reminds us that we can still love and be loved

When we feel gripped by rage, hope is not far away

When we must say goodbye to those we love, hope reminds us the best is yet to come.

Hope is measurable. Hope is malleable. Hope can rise. Spread the word.

About the Authors

Casey Gwinn, J.D.

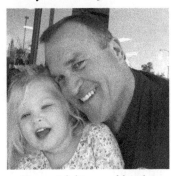

Casey with his granddaughter

Casey Gwinn serves as the President of Alliance for HOPE International—one of the leading systems and social change organizations in the country focused on creating collaborative, trauma-informed approaches to meeting the needs of survivors of domestic violence and sexual assault and their children. He is the former elected City Attorney of San Diego and the visionary behind the rapidly developing international Family Justice Center movement—bringing together, under one roof, services to victims of domestic violence, sexual assault, and stalking and their children. He has been recognized as one of the top 45 public lawyers in America.

Casey is the founder of the nationally recognized Camp HOPE America, the first evidence-based camping and mentoring program focused on children exposed to domestic violence. He has authored or co-authored ten books and hundreds of articles and media commentaries.

He has been profiled in news outlets in the United States including The Huffington Post, the New York Times, the New Yorker, ABC Nightly News, CNN, The Early Show on CBS, and the Oprah Winfrey Show.

Casey lives in San Diego with his wife Beth. He has three grown children and three grandchildren.

Chan M. Hellman, PhD.

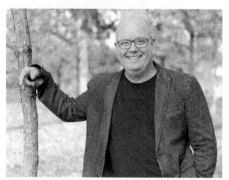

Photo courtesy of Callen Vo

Chan is a professor in the Anne & Henry Zarrow School of Social Work and Founding Director of The Hope Research Center at the University of Oklahoma. Chan holds Adjunct Professor appointments in the Department of Internal Medicine and Department of Pediatrics for the OU College of Medicine and the Department of Health Promotion Sciences for the OU College of Public Health. He has written more than 150 scientific publications and has presented at numerous national and international conferences worldwide. Chan's research is focused on hope as a psychological strength helping children and adults overcome trauma and adversity.

Chan teaches master's and doctoral level students primarily in the areas of positive psychology, research methods, and statistics. He also directs student research in the areas of hope and nonprofit organizations.

Chan is a lifelong Oklahoman, and lives in Tulsa Oklahoma with his wife Kendra. They enjoy spending time with their children and grandchildren, traveling, and reading.

Acknowledgements

It is almost impossible to thank everyone who made this book possible. We want to thank Chan's graduate students—Rachel Baluh and Jason Featherngill—for their help in the research cited in this book and assistance with proofreading and editing along with Ric Munoz and Shawn Schaefer and other faculty members at The University of Oklahoma's Hope Research Center. Thank you to Suzann Stewart at the Tulsa Family Safety Center for introducing us to each other in 2012. She changed the destinies of our lives. Dr. Joseph Bellezzo at Sharp Memorial Hospital helped us immensely with the opening story of the book. We are committed to helping him spread the word about ED ECMO and saving lives in hospitals around the world. We are deeply indebted to our wives, Beth (Casey) and Kendra (Chan), for their support, feedback, editing, and patience in the emotionally draining and time-consuming journey of writing. Special thanks to Karen Anderson, David Hancock, Margo Toulouse, and the team at Morgan James Publishing for believing in this book and its message.

The entire staff at Alliance for HOPE International has been part of this in small and large ways. CEO Gael Strack has helped us in writing, editing, and framing. She is such a gifted leader and writer in her own right and her leadership has been crucial to the success of our work and research around hope. The Alliance's Polyvictimization Team, Natalia Aguirre, Alison Bildsoe, and Gloria Kyallo, is doing such amazing work with Family Justice Centers across the country and their research and work has allowed us to think deeply about trauma-informed care and hope-centered work with victims of trauma. Special thanks to Natalia Aguirre and Maddie Orcutt for being excellent content editors and Karianne Johansen for her research, writing, and editing for us around nutrition and brain-body modalities.

Thank you to Michael Burke for his leadership of Camp HOPE America and all those across the country that have joined us in the vision for working with high ACE Score children and teens. We appreciate the entire Camp HOPE America team for their world-changing work—Maddie Orcutt, Karianne Johansen, Chelsea Armstrong, and Melissa Aguiar. Special thanks to Carrie Hughes at Verizon for investing so much time, passion, and heart in the expansion of Camp HOPE America. Thank you to the Board of the Alliance for their support—Bob Martin, Gil Cabrera, Mike Scogin, Lilys McCoy, and Jerry Fineman. Thank you as well to those who don't often get noticed at the Alliance but are doing such hope giving work day in and day out—Sarah Sherman Julien, Sarah Dillon, Jenny Dietzen, Gemma Serrano, and Yolanda Ruiz.

We also want to acknowledge Stacy Phillips and Susan Williams at the U.S. Department of Justice, Office for Victims of Crime for developing a national polyvictimization initiative that has informed our thinking about working with adult and child survivors.

We honor Lucia Corral-Pena and the Blue Shield of California Foundation for supporting our development of the Family Justice Center movement in California including our research on the power of the hope in the lives of survivors.

Thank you to the Charles and Lynn Schusterman Foundation in Tulsa who have supported our call for hope-centered outcome evaluation in nonprofit organizations. They sponsored the first Nonprofits as Pathways of Hope Conference in Oklahoma and became the first major funder to call for measuring hope everywhere.

We want to recognize the leadership of Carrie Hughes at the Verizon Foundation for supporting our work with Camp HOPE America. Rose Kirk, Mike Mason, Carrie, and many others at Verizon have invested so heavily over the years in helping domestic violence survivors and their children. Carrie challenged us as much as anyone ever has to measure our results including measuring hope and related outcomes. She took us to a whole new level in our work.

Special thanks to Yesenia Aceves, the Director of the Pathways program of Camp HOPE America, for her work in proving that rising hope can be sustained all year long and year after year in the lives of trauma survivors if we invest the time and energy to build a community of hope and support. Yesenia is also a gifted graphic artist and helped with the graphics of the book and all our Hope Scales.

Most of all we thank the courageous women, men, and young people who shared their stories with us for this book. They are the true hope heroes. All the stories in the book are true because they told the truth about their lives, struggles, and successes and inspired us to do the same.

Sample Domains of HOPE

THE ACADEMIC DOMAIN

Directions: Read each sentence carefully. For each sentence, please think about how you are in most situations. Using the scale shown below, please select the number that best describes **YOU** the best and put that number in the blank provided. There are no right or wrong answers.

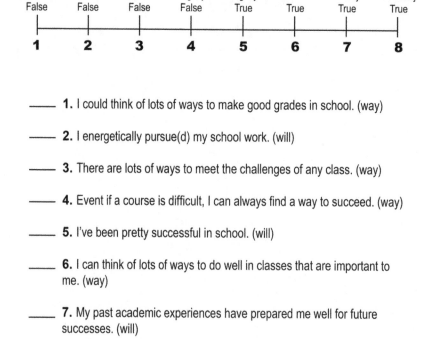

Definitely False	Mostly False	Somewhat False	Slightly False	Slightly True	Somewhat True	Mostly True	Definitely True
1	2	3	4	5	6	7	8

_____ **1.** I could think of lots of ways to make good grades in school. (way)

_____ **2.** I energetically pursue(d) my school work. (will)

_____ **3.** There are lots of ways to meet the challenges of any class. (way)

_____ **4.** Event if a course is difficult, I can always find a way to succeed. (way)

_____ **5.** I've been pretty successful in school. (will)

_____ **6.** I can think of lots of ways to do well in classes that are important to me. (way)

_____ **7.** My past academic experiences have prepared me well for future successes. (will)

_____ **8.** I got the grades I wanted in my classes. (will)

THE HEALTH AND FITNESS DOMAIN

Directions: Read each sentence carefully. For each sentence, please think about how you are in most situations. Using the scale shown below, please select the number that best describes **YOU** and put that number in the blank provided. There are no right or wrong answers.

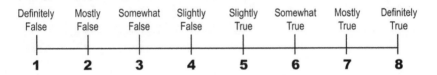

Definitely False	Mostly False	Somewhat False	Slightly False	Slightly True	Somewhat True	Mostly True	Definitely True
1	2	3	4	5	6	7	8

_____ **1.** I can think many ways to maintain my health and fitness. (way)

_____ **2.** I actively work at being healthy and fit. (will)

_____ **3.** Even when I am tired, I can usually make myself work out. (will)

_____ **4.** I can find ways to continue my health and fitness routines in a variety of situations (e.g., traveling). (way)

_____ **5.** I believe I can sustain my health and fitness as I grow older. (will)

_____ **6.** Habits of health and fitness I acquired in the past will help me in the future. (way)

THE FAMILY DOMAIN

Directions: Read each sentence carefully. For each sentence, please think about how you are in most situations. Using the scale shown below, please select the number that best describes **YOU** and put that number in the blank provided. There are no right or wrong answers.

Definitely False	Mostly False	Somewhat False	Slightly False	Slightly True	Somewhat True	Mostly True	Definitely True
1	2	3	4	5	6	7	8

_____ **1.** I can think of lots of things I enjoy doing with my family. (way)

_____ **2.** I energetically work on maintaining family relationships. (will)

_____ **3.** I can think of many ways to include my family in things that are important to me. (way)

_____ **4.** I have a pretty successful family life. (will)

_____ **5.** Even when we disagree, I know my family can find a way to solve our problems. (way)

_____ **6.** I have the kid of relationships that I want with family members. (will)

_____ **7.** There are lots of ways to communicate my feelings to family members. (way)

_____ **8.** My own experiences with family have prepared me for a family of my own. (will)

THE DOMAIN OF ROMANTIC RELATIONSHIPS

Directions: Read each sentence carefully. For each sentence, please think about how you are in most situations. Using the scale shown below, please select the number that best describes **YOU** and put that number in the blank provided. There are no right or wrong answers.

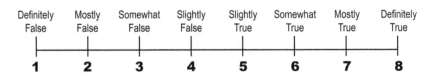

Definitely False	Mostly False	Somewhat False	Slightly False	Slightly True	Somewhat True	Mostly True	Definitely True
1	2	3	4	5	6	7	8

_____ **1.** I can think many ways to get to know someone to whom I am attracted. (way)

_____ **2.** When I'm interested in someone romantically, I actively pursue them. (will)

_____ **3.** I've been pretty successful in my romantic relationships. (will)

_____ **4.** There are lots of ways to convince someone to go out with me. (way)

_____ **5.** I can think of many ways to keep someone interested in me when they are important. (way)

_____ **6.** My past romantic relationships have prepared me well for future involvements. (way)

_____ **7.** Even when someone doesn't seem interested, I know I can get their attention. (will)

_____ **8.** I can usually get a date when I set my mind to it. (will)

References

(Provided in Order of Appearance)

Introduction

1. Snyder, C. R. (2000). *Handbook of hope: Theory, measures, and applications.* San Diego, CA: Academic Press.

2. Lopez, S. J. (2014). *Making hope happen: Creating the future you want for yourself and others.* New York City, NY: Atria books.

3. Karr-Morse, R. (2013). *Ghosts from the nursery: Tracing the roots of violence.* New York City, NY: Atlantic Monthly Press.

4. Karr-Morese, R. (2012). *Scared sick: The role of childhood trauma in adult disease.* New York City, NY: Basic Books.

5. Felitti, V. J., Anda, R. F., Nordenberg, D., Williamson, D. F., Spitz, A. M., Edwards, V., Koss, M. P., & Marks, J. S. (1998). Relationship of childhood abuse and household dysfunction to many of the leading causes of death in adults: The Adverse Childhood Experiences (ACE) study. *American Journal of Preventative Medicine, 14,* 245-258.

6. Besser van der Kolk (2014). *The body keeps the score: brain, mind, and body in the healing of trauma.* New York, NY: Penguin Books.

7. Brown, B. (2012). *Daring greatly: How the courage to be vulnerable transforms the way we live, love, parent, and lead.* New York City, NY: Avery.

8.   Brown, B. (2017). *Braving the wilderness: The quest for true belonging and the courage to stand alone.* New York, NY: Penguin Books.

9.   Burke Harris, N. (2018). *The Deepest Well: Healing the Long-Term Effects of Childhood Adversity.* Boston, MA: Houghton Mifflin Harcourt

10.   Gwinn, C. (2015). *Cheering for the Children: Creating Pathways to HOPE for Children Exposed to Trauma.* Tucson, AZ: Wheatmark Press.

Chapter 2: What is Hope?

11.   Snyder, C. R. (2000). *Handbook of hope: Theory, measures, and applications.* San Diego, CA: Academic Press.

12.   Snyder, C. R. (2002). Hope theory: Rainbows in the mind. *Psychological Inquiry, 13,* 249-275.

13.   Gailliot, M. T., & Baumeister, R. F. (2016). The physiology of willpower: Linking blood glucose to self-control. *Personality and Social Psychology Review, 11,* 303-327.

14.   Magaletta, P. R., & Oliver, M. M. (1999). The hope construct, will and ways: Their relative relations with self-efficacy, optimism, and general well-being. *Journal of Clinical Psychology, 55,* 539-551.

15.   De Becker, G. (1997). The gift of fear: Survival signals that protect us from violence. New York City: NY: Dell.

Chapter 3: Why Hope Matters So Much

16.   Park, N., Peterson, C., & Seligman, M. E. P. (2004). Strengths of character and well-being. *Journal of Social and Clinical Psychology, 23,* 603-619.

17.   Snyder, C. R. (2004). Hope and other strengths: Lessons from Animal Farm. *Journal of Social and Clinical Psychology, 23,* 624-627.

18.   Marques, S. C., Lopez, S. J., & Pais-Ribeiro, J. L. (2011). Building hope for the future: A program to foster strengths in middle-school students. *Journal of Happiness Studies, 12,* 139-152.

19.   Marques, S. C., Gallagher, M. W., & Lopez, S. J. (2017). Hope and academic-related outcomes: A meta-analysis. *School Mental Health, 9,* 250-262.

20.   Gallagher, M. W., Marques, S. C., & Lopez, S. J. (2017). Hope and academic trajectory of college students. *Journal of Happiness Studies, 18,* 341-352.

21. Brooks, D. (2012). *The psych approach*. New York Times. Available on-line: http://www.nytimes.com/2012/09/28/opinion/brooks-the-psych-approach.html

22. Gallup. (2013). *Measuring hope, engagement, and well-being of America's students*. Available on-line: http://www.gallup.com/services/176723/measuring-hope-engagement-wellbeing-america-students.aspx

23. Reichard, R. J., Avey, J. B., Lopez, S. J., & Dollwet, M. (2013). Having the will and finding the way: A review and meta-analysis of hope at work. *The Journal of Positive Psychology, 8*, 292-304.

24. Simmons, B. L., Gooty, J., Nelson, D. L., & Little, L. M. (2009). Secure attachment: Implications for hope, trust, burnout, and performance. *Journal of Organizational Behavior, 30*, 233-247.

25. Groopman, J. (2004). *The anatomy of hope: How people prevail in the face of illness*. New York, NY: Radom House.

26. Allen, J. V., Steele, R. G., Nelson, M. B., Peugh, J., Egan, A., Clements, M., & Patton, S. R. (2016). A longitudinal examination of hope and optimism and their role in Type 1 diabetes in youths. *Journal of Pediatric Psychology, 41*, 741-749.

27. Lloyd, S. M., Cantell, M., Pacaud, D., Crawford, S., & Dewey, D. (2009). Brief report: Hope, perceived maternal empathy, medical regimen adherence, and glycemic control in adolescents with Type 1 diabetes. *Journal of Pediatric Psychology, 34*, 1025-1029.

28. Mednick, L., Cogen, F., Henderson, C., Rohrbeck, C. A., Kitessa, D., & Streisand, R. (2007). Hope more, worry less: Hope as a potential resilience factor in mothers of very young children with Type 1 diabetes. *Children's Healthcare, 36*, 385-396.

29. Tse, S., Murray, G., Chung, K. F., Davidson, L., Ng K. L., Yu, CH. (2014). Exploring the recovery concept in bipolar disorder: A decision tree analysis of psychosocial correlates of recovery stages. *Bipolar Disorders, 16*, 366-377.

30. Oles, S. K., Fukui, S., Rand, K. L., & Salyers, M. P. (2015). The relationship between hope and patient activation in consumers with schizophrenia: Results from longitudinal analyses. *Psychiatry Research, 228*, 272-276.

31. Werner, S. (2012). Subjective well-being, hope, and needs of individuals with serious mental illness. *Psychiatry Research, 196*, 214-219.

32. Kylma, J., Juvakka, T., Nikkonen, M., Korhonen, T., & Isohanni, M. (2006). Hope and schizophrenia: An integrative review. *Journal of Psychiatric and Mental Health Nursing, 13*, 651-664.

33. Park, J., & Chen, R. K. (2016). Positive psychology and hope as a means to recovery from mental illness. *Journal of Applied Rehabilitation Counseling, 47*, 34-42.

34. Snyder, C. R. (2000). *Handbook of hope: Theory, measures, and applications.* San Diego, CA: Academic Press.

35. Munoz, T. R., Bull, L., Sheth, D., Gower, S., Engstrom, E., Brunk, K., Hellman, C. M., & Fox, M. D. (2014). The predictive power of Adverse Childhood Experiences on trust in the medical profession among residents of a public housing facility. *Annals of Community Medicine and Practice, 1*, 995-1002.

36. Elliott, T. R., Witty, T. E., Herrick, S., & Hoffman, J. T. (1991). Negotiating reality after physical loss: Hope, depression, and disability. *Journal of Personality and Social Psychology, 61*, 608-613.

37. Parashar, D. (2015). The trajectory of hope: Pathways to finding meaning and reconstructing the self after a spinal cord injury. *Spinal Cord, 53*, 565-568.

38. Yadav, S. (2010). Perceived social support, hope, and quality of life of persons living with HIV/AIDS: A case study from Nepal. *Quality of Life Research, 19*, 157-166.

39. Berendes, D., Keefe, F. J., Somers, T. J., Kothadia, S. M., Porter, L. S., & Cheavens, J. S. (2010). Hope in the context of lung cancer: Relationships of hope to symptoms and psychological distress. *Journal of Pain and Symptom Management, 40*, 174-182.

Chapter 4: Telling the Truth About Your Life

40. Snyder, C. R. (2000). *Handbook of hope: Theory, measures, and applications.* San Diego, CA: Academic Press.

41. Snyder, C. R. (2002). Hope theory: Rainbows in the mind. *Psychological Inquiry, 13*, 249-275.

42. Bessel van der Kolk (2014). *The body keeps the score: brain, mind, and body in the healing of trauma.* New York, NY: Penguin Books.

43. Frederickson, B. (2009). *Positivity: Top-notch research reveals the upward spiral that will change your life.* New York City, NY: Harmony Books.

Chapter 5: Hope Should Be Measured Everywhere

44.   Snyder, C. R., Berg, C., Woodward, J. T., Gum, A., Randk, K. L., Wrobleski, K. K., Brown, J., & Hackman, A. (2005). Hope against the cold: Individual differences in trait hope and acute pain tolerance on the cold pressor task. *Journal of Personality, 73*, 287-312.

45.   Snyder, C. R., Harris, D., Anderson, J. R., Holleran, S. A., Irving, L. M., Sigmon, S. T., Yoshinobu, L., Gibb, J., Langelle, C., & Harney, P. (1991). The will and the ways: Development and validation of an individual-differences measure of hope. *Journal of Personality and Social Psychology, 60*, 570-585.

46.   Snyder, C. R., Hoza, B., Pelham, W. E., Rapoff, M., Ware, L., Danovsky, M., Highberger, L., Rubinstein, H., & Stahl, K. J. (1997). The development and validation of the Children's Hope Scale. *Journal of Pediatric Psychology, 22*, 399-421.

47.   Sympson, S. C. (1999). *Validation of the domain specific hope scale: Exploring hope in life domains.* Unpublished Dissertation. University of Kansas.

48.   Hellman, C. M., Pittman, M. K., & Munoz, R. T. (2013). The first twenty years of the will and the ways: An examination of score reliability distribution on Snyder's Dispositional Hope Scale. *Journal of Happiness Studies, 14*, 723-729.

49.   Hellman, C. M., Munoz, R. T., Worley, J. A., Feeley, J. A., & Gillert, J. E. (In Press). A reliability generalization on the Children's Hope Scale. *Child Indicators Research.*

Chapter 6: Measuring Hope in Children and Teens

50.   Snyder, C. R., Hoza, B., Pelham, W. E., Rapoff, M., Ware, L., Danovsky, M., Highberger, L., Rubinstein, H., & Stahl, K. J. (1997). The development and validation of the Children's Hope Scale. *Journal of Pediatric Psychology, 22*, 399-421.

51.   Hellman, C. M., Munoz, R. T., Worley, J. A., Feeley, J. A., & Gillert, J. E. (In Press). A reliability generalization on the Children's Hope Scale. *Child Indicators Research.*

52.   Hellman, C. M. & Gwinn, C. (2017). Children exposed to domestic violence: Examining the effects of Camp HOPE on children's hope, resilience, and strength of character. *Child and Adolescent Social Work Journal, 34*, 269-276.

53.   Pedrotti, J. T., Edwards, L., & Lopez, S. J. (2008). Promoting hope: Suggestions for school counselors. *Professional School Counseling, 12*, 100-107.

Chapter 9: The Adverse Childhood Experiences (ACE) Study

54.   Baxter, M. A., Hemming, E. J., McIntosh, H. C., & Hellman, C. M. (2017). Exploring the relationship between adverse childhood experiences and hope. *The Journal of Child Sexual Abuse, 8*, 948-956.

55.   Fry-Grier, L., & Hellman, C. M. (2017). School aged children of incarcerated parents: The effects of alternative criminal sentencing. *Child Indicators Research, 10*, 859-879.

56.   Hellman, C. M. & Gwinn, C. (2017). Children exposed to domestic violence: Examining the effects of Camp HOPE on children's hope, resilience, and strength of character. *Child and Adolescent Social Work Journal, 34*, 269-276.

57.   Munoz, R.T., Brunk, K., & Hellman, C. M. (In Press). The relationship between hope, self-efficacy, and life satisfaction among a sample of survivors of intimate partner violence. *The Journal of Applied Quality of Life.*

58.   Muñoz, R.T., Hellman, C. M., Buster, B., Robbins, A., Carroll, C. Kabbani, M., Cassody, L., Brahm, N., & Fox, M. (2016). Life satisfaction, hope, and positive emotions as antecedents of health related quality of life among homeless individuals. *International Journal of Applied Positive Psychology. 1, 69-89.*

59.   Munoz, T. R., Bull, L., Sheth, D., Gower, S., Engstrom, E., Brunk, K., Hellman, C. M., Fox, M. (2014). The predictive power of Adverse Childhood Experiences on Trust in the Medical Profession among residents of a public housing facility. *Annals of Community Medicine and Practice. 1*, 995-1002.

60.   Felitti, V. J., Anda, R. F., Nordenberg, D., Williamson, D. F., Spitz, A. M., Edwards, V., Koss, M. P., & Marks, J. S. (1998). Relationship of childhood abuse and household dysfunction to many of the leading causes of death in adults: The Adverse Childhood Experiences (ACE) study. *American Journal of Preventative Medicine, 14*, 245-258.

61.   Center for Disease Control. *Adverse Childhood Experiences.* Available online at: https://www.cdc.gov/violenceprevention/acestudy/index.html.

62. Anda, R. F., Brown, D. W., Felitti, V. J., Dube, S. R., & Giles, W. H. (2008). Adverse childhood experiences and prescription drug use in a cohort study of adult HMO patients. *BMC Public Health, 8,* 198-206.

63. Lassri, D., & Shahar, G. (2012). Self-criticism mediates the link between childhood emotional maltreatment and young adults' romantic relationships. *Journal of Social and Clinical Psychology, 31,* 289-311.

64. Lassri, D., Luyten, P., Cohen, G., & Sharar, G. (2016). The effect of childhood emotional maltreatment on romantic relationships in young adulthood: A double mediation model involving self-criticism and attachment. *Psychological Trauma: Theory, Research, Practice, and Policy, 8,* 504-511.

65. Wolff, N., & Shi, J. (2012). Childhood and adult trauma experiences of incarcerated persons and their relationship to adult behavioral health problems and treatment. *International Journal of Environmental Research and Public Health, 9,* 1908-1926.

66. Cuadra, L. E., Jaffe, A. E., Thomas, R., & Dilillo, D. (2014). Child maltreatment and adult criminal behavior: Does criminal thinking explain the association? *Child Abuse & Neglect,* 38, 1399-1408.

67. Bride, B. E., Hatcher, S. S., & Humble, M. N. (2009). Trauma training, trauma practices, and secondary traumatic stress among substance abuse counselors. *Traumatology, 15,* 96-105.

68. Munoz, R. T., Brady, S., & Brown, V. (2017). The psychology of resilience: A model of the relationship of locus of control to hope among survivors of intimate partner violence. *Traumatology, 23,* 102-111.

69. National Scientific Council on the Developing Child (2010). Early experiences can alter gene expression and affect long-term development: Working Paper No. 10. http://www.develpingchild.net.

Chapter 10: Sometimes It is Too Late for Hope

70. Strack, G., Gwinn, C. (eds.) (2014). *Domestic Violence Report,* Vol. 19, No. 6. Available online at: https://www.familyjusticecenter.org/wp-content/uploads/2017/11/Civic-Research-Institute-Domestic-Violence-Report-a-Special-Issue-on-Strangulation-2014.pdf.

Chapter 11: Great Leader, Visionaries, and Gifted People with Demons

71. Dube, S.R., Anda, R.F., Felitti, V.J., et al (2001). Childhood abuse, household dysfunction, and the risk of attempted suicide throughout the

lifespan; findings from the Adverse Childhood Experiences Study. *Journal of the American Medical Association*, 286 (24); 3089-96.

72.   World Health Organization (2017). Suicide data. Available on-line at: http://www.who.int/mental_health/prevention/suicide/suicideprevent/en/

73.   LeardMann, C. A., Powell, T. M., Smith, T. C., Bell, M. R., Smith, B., Boyko, E. J., Hooper, T. I., Gackstetter, G. D., Ghamsary, M., & Hoge, C. W. (2013). Risk factors associated with suicide in current and former US military personnel. *Journal of America Medical Association, 310*, 496-506.

74.   Ensler, E. (2008). *The vagina monologues*. New York, NY: Villard Books.

75.   Snyder, C. R., (2004). Hope and depression: A light in the darkness. *Journal of Social and Clinical Psychology, 23*, 347-351.

76.   Chapman, D. P., Whitfield, C. L., Felitti, V. J., Dube, S. R., & Anda, R. F. (2004). Adverse childhood experiences and the risk of depressive disorders in adulthood. *Journal of Affective Disorders, 15*, 217-225.

77.   Arnau, R. C., Rosen, D. H., Finch, J. F., Rhudy, J. L., & Fortunato, V. J. (2007). Longitudinal effects of hope on depression and anxiety: A latent variable analysis. *Journal of Personality, 75*, 43-64.

78.   Brueck, H., *Business Insider.* (2017). Available online at: http://www.businessinsider.com/deadliest-mass-shootings-almost-all-have-domestic-violence-connection-2017-11.

Chapter 12: Lessons Learned from Abused Kids

79.   Hellman, C. M., Robinson-Keilig, R. A., Dubriwny, N. M., Hamil, C., & Kraft, A. (In Press). Hope as a coping resource for parents at-risk for child abuse and neglect. *Journal of Family Social Work*.

80.   Hellman, C. M., & Gwinn, C. (2017). Children exposed to domestic violence: Examining the effects of Camp HOPE on children's hope, resilience, and strength of character. *Child and Adolescent Social Work Journal, 34*, 269-276.

81.   Gwinn, C. (2015). *Cheering for the Children: Creating Pathways to HOPE for Children Exposed to Trauma.* Tucson, AZ: Wheatmark Press.

Chapter 13: Lessons Learned from Battered Women

82.   Gwinn, C., & Strack, G. (2010). *Dream big: A simple, complicated idea to stop family violence.* Tucson, AZ: Wheatmark Press.

83.   Hellman, C. M., Gwinn, C., Strack, G., Burke, M., Featherngill, J., Aguirre, N., & Aceves, Y. (2017). Survivor defined success, hope, and well-

being: An assessment of the impact of Family Justice Centers. Available on-line at: https://www.familyjusticecenter.org/media/media-releases/.

84. Munoz, R.T., Brunk, K., & Hellman, C. M. (2017). The relationship between hope and life satisfaction among survivors of intimate partner violence: The enhancing effect of self-efficacy. *Applied Research in Quality of Life, 12,* 981-995.

Chapter 14: Hope and the Human Brain

85. Gallup World Poll (2013). Findings available on-line at: http://news.gallup.com/topic/world_region_worldwide.aspx

86. Gottschalk, L., Fronczek, J., & Buchsbaum, M. (1993). The cerebral neurobiology of hope and hopelessness. *Psychiatry, 56,* 270-281.

87. Lisak, D. (2013). The neurobiology of trauma. Available on-line at: https://www.nccpsafety.org/resources/library/the-neurobiology-of-trauma/

88. Burke Harris, N (2015). How childhood trauma affects health across a lifetime. Available on-line at: https://www.ted.com/talks/nadine_burke_harris_how_childhood_trauma_affects_health_across_a_lifetime

89. Lucado, M. (2017). *Anxious for nothing: Finding calm in a chaotic world.* Nashville, TN: Harper Collins Publishers.

90. National Institute of Mental Health. (nd). Any anxiety disorder among adults. Report available on-line at: https://www.nimh.nih.gov/health/statistics/prevalence/any-anxiety-disorder-among-adults.shtml

91. World Health Organization. (2017). Depression and other common mental health disorders. (WHO Ref. WHO/MSD/MER/2017.2).

92. de Becker, G. (1998). *The gift of fear: Survival signals that protect us from violence.* New York, NY: Little, Brown & Company.

93. Ong, A. D., Edwards, L. M., & Bergeman, C. S. (2006). Hope as a source of resilience in later adulthood. *Personality and Individual Differences, 41,* 1263-1273.

94. Whippman, R. (2016). *America the anxious: How our pursuit of happiness is creating a nation of nervous wrecks.* New York City, NY: St. Martin's Press.

95. Lopez, S. J. (2014). *Making hope happen: Creating the future you want for yourself and others.* New York City, NY: Atria books.

96. Ford, J. D., Racusin, R., Ellis, C. G., Davis, W. B., Reiser, J., Fleischer, A., & Thomas, J. (2000). Child maltreatment, other trauma exposure, and posttraumatic symptomatology among children with oppositional defiant

and attention deficit hyperactivity disorders. *Child Maltreatment, 5,* 205-217.

97. Ruiz, R. (2014). How childhood trauma could be mistaken for ADHD. The Atlantic (June 7, 2014). Available on-line at: www.theatlantic.com/health/archive/2014/07/how-childhood-trauma-could-be-mistaken-for-adhd/373328/.

98. Szymanski, K., Sapanski, L., & Conway, F. (2011). Trauma and ADHD—association or diagnostic confusion? A clinical perspective. *Journal of infant, Child & Adolescent Psychotherapy, 10,* 51-59.

99. Levine, P. A. (2015). *Trauma and memory: Brain and body in a search for the living past: A practical guide for understanding and working with traumatic memory.* Berkley, CA: North Atlantic Books.

100. Brom, D., Stokar, Y., Lawi, C., Nuriel-Porat, V., Ziv, Y., Lerner, K., & Ross, G. (2017). Somatic experiencing for posttraumatic stress disorder: A randomized controlled outcome study. *Journal of Traumatic Stress, 30,* 304-312.

101. Chamberlain L. (2016). *Assessment Tools for Children's Exposure to Violence.* Defending Childhood Initiative, Futures Without Violence. Available on-line at: http://promising.futureswithoutviolence.org/files/2012/01/Assessment-Tools-for-Childrens-Exposure-to-Violence-2016.pdf

102. Doidge, N. (2015). *The brain's way of healing: Remarkable discoveries and recoveries from the frontiers of neuroplasticity.* New York, NY: Penguin Books.

103. Bessel van der Kolk (2014). *The body keeps the score: brain, mind, and body in the healing of trauma.* New York, NY: Penguin Books.

104. Hoppes, S. Bryce, H., Hellman, C. M., & Finlay, E. (2012). The effects of brief mindfulness training on caregivers' well-being. *Activities, Adaptation, & Aging, 36,* 147-166.

105. Munoz, R.T., Hoppes, S., Hellman, C.M., Brunk, K.L., Bragg, J.E., & Cummins, C. (In Press). The effects of mindfulness meditation on hope and stress. *Research on Social Work Practice.*

106. Campbell, J. C., Anderson, J. C., McFadgion, A., Gill, J., Zink, E., Patch, M., Callwood, G., & Campbell, D. (2017). The effects of intimate partner violence and brain injury on central nervous system symptoms. *Journal of Women's Health.* https://doi.org/10.1089/jwh.2016.6311.

Chapter 15: Illness, Nutrition, and Hope

107.	Macon, R. K. (2014). *Feeding hope through Tulsa's philanthropic community.* Unpublished Dissertation, University of Oklahoma.

108.	Kritharis, A., Pilichowska, M., & Evens, A. M. (2016). How I manage patients with grey zone lymphoma. *British Journal of Haematology, 174,* 345-350.

109.	Munoz, R.T., Hoppes, S., Hellman, C.M., Brunk, K.L., Bragg, J.E., & Cummins, C. (In Press). The effects of mindfulness meditation on hope and stress. *Research on Social Work Practice.*

110.	Sears, S., & Kraus, S. (2009). I think therefore I am: Cognitive distortions and coping style as mediators for the effects of mindfulness meditation on anxiety, positive and negative affect, and hope. *Journal of Clinical Psychology, 65,* 561-573.

111.	Crothers, M. K., Tomter, H. D., & Garske, J. P. (2005). The relationships between satisfaction with social support, affect balance, and hope in cancer patients. *Journal of Psychosocial Oncology, 23,* 103-118.

112.	Toles, M., Dmark-Wahnefried, W. (2008). Nutrition and the cancer survivor: Evidence to guide oncology nursing practice. *Seminars in Oncology Nursing, 24,* 171-179.

113.	Haelle, T. (2017). Hope comes in many forms for patients with cancer: For many with glioblastoma, there's no clear path after standard therapy, but scientists are exploring an array of new options. *CURE: Cancer Updates, Research & Education, 16,* 1-7.

114.	Wright, J. V., & Lenard, L. (2001). *Why stomach acid is good for you: Natural relief from heartburn, indigestion, reflux & GERD.* Lanham, MD: M. Evans & Company.

115.	Martin, G. R. R. (2011). *A game of thrones.* New York City, NY: Bantam Books.

Chapter 17: Teaching to the Test (aka Studying the Answers)

116.	Hellman, C. M., & Gwinn, C. (2017). Children exposed to domestic violence: Examining the effects of Camp HOPE on children's hope, resilience, and strength of character. *Child and Adolescent Social Work Journal, 34,* 269-276.

117.	Snyder, C. R., (1995). Conceptualizing, measuring, and nurturing hope. *Journal of Counseling & Development, 73,* 355-360.

118.	Angelou, M. (1978). *And still I rise.* New York, NY: Random House.

119. Emmons, R. A., & Stern, R. (2013). Gratitude as a psychotherapeutic intervention. *Journal of Clinical Psychology: In Session, 69*, 846-855.

120. Emmons, R. A., & McCullough, M. E. (2004). *The psychology of gratitude.* New York, NY: Oxford University Press.

121. Peterson, C., & Seligman, M. E. P. (2004). *Character strengths and virtues: A handbook and classification.* New York, NY: Oxford University Press.

122. Smalley, G., & Trent, J. (1990). *The blessing.* New York City, NY: Pocket Books.

123. Bessel van der Kolk (2014). *The body keeps the score: brain, mind, and body in the healing of trauma.* New York, NY: Penguin Books.

124. Saleebey, D. (2000). Power in the people: Strengths and hope. *Advances in Social Work, 1,* 127-136.

125. Gwinn, C. (2015). *Cheering for the Children: Creating Pathways to HOPE for Children Exposed to Trauma.* Tucson, AZ: Wheatmark Press.

126. Chaturvedi, S., Arvey, R. d., Zhang, Z., & Chsritoforou, P. T. (2011). Genetic underpinnings of transformational leadership: The mediation role of dispositional hope. *Journal of Leadership & Organizational Studies, 18,* 469-479.

127. Sulimani-Aidan, Y. (2017). Future expectations as a source of resilience among young people leaving care. *British Journal of Social Work, 47,* 1111-1127.

Chapter 18: Spirituality and Hope

128. Pew Research Center (2014). *Religious landscape study.* Available on-line at: http://www.pewforum.org/religious-landscape-study/

129. Ellison, C. G., & Levin, J. S. (1998). The religion-health connection: Evidence, theory, and future directions. *Health Education & Behavior, 25,* 700-720.

130. McIntosh, D. N., Poulin, M. J., Silver, R. C., & Holman, E. A. (2011). The distinct roles of spirituality and religiosity in physical and mental health after collective trauma: A national longitudinal study of responses to the 9/11 attacks. *Journal of Behavioral Medicine, 34,* 497-507.

131. Bryant-Davis, T., & Wong, E. C. (2013). Faith to move mountains: Religious coping, spirituality, and interpersonal trauma recovery. *American Psychologist, 68,* 675-684.

132. Smith, S. (2004). Exploring the interaction of trauma and spirituality. *Traumatology, 10,* 231-243.

133. Kübler-Ross, E. (1969). *On Death and dying: What the dying have to teach doctors, nurses, clergy, and their own families.* New York, NY: The Macmillan Company.

134. Marques, S. C., Lopez, S. J., & Mitchell, J. (2013). The role of hope, spirituality and religious practice in adolescents' life satisfaction: Longitudinal findings. *Journal of Happiness Studies, 14,* 251-261.

135. Lyubomirsky, S. (2007). *The how of happiness: A new approach to getting the life you want.* New York, NY: Penguin Books.

Chapter 19: Pursuing a Hope-Centered Life

136. Seuss, D. (1990). *Oh the places you'll go!* New York, NY: Random House.

137. Feldman, D. B., Dreher, D. E. (2012). Can hope be changed in 90 minutes? Testing the efficacy of a single-session goal-pursuit intervention for college students. *Journal of Happiness Studies, 13,* 745-759.

138. Snyder, C. R., Rand, K. L., King, E. A., Feldman, D. B., & Woodward, J. T. (2002). False hope. *Journal of Clinical Psychology, 58,* 1003-1022.

Chapter 20: The Hope-Centered Workplace

139. Gallup, Inc. (2017). *State of the American workplace.* Retrieved from: http://news.gallup.com/reports/199961/7.aspx

140. Rath, T., & Conchie, B. (2009). *Strengths based leadership: Great leaders, teams, and why people follow.* Omaha, NE: Gallup Press.

141. Peale, M. V. (2003). *The power of positive thinking.* New York, NY: Touchstone.

142. Seligman, M. E. P., & Csikszentmihalyi, M. (2000). Positive psychology: An introduction. *American Psychologist, 55,* 5-14.

143. Seligman, M. E. P. (2011). *Flourish.* New York, NY: Free Press.

144. Peterson, C. (2008). What is positive psychology, and what is it not? Psychology Today, available on-line at: https://www.psychologytoday.com/blog/the-good-life/200805/what-is-positive-psychology-and-what-is-it-not

145. Luthans, F., Luthans, K. W., & Luthans, B. C. (2004). Positive psychological capital: Beyond human and social capital. *Business Horizons, 47,* 45-50.

146. Youssef, C. M., & Luthans, F. (2007). Positive organizational behavior in the workplace: The impact of hope, optimism, and resilience. *Journal of Management, 33,* 774-800.

147.   Jenkins, S. R., & Baird, S. (2002). Secondary traumatic stress and vicarious trauma: A validational study. *Journal of Traumatic Stress, 15*, 423-432.

148.   Figley, C. R. (2002). *Treating compassion fatigue.* New York, NY: Brunner-Routledge.

149.   Maslach, C. (1982). *Burnout: The cost of caring.* Englewood Cliffs, NJ: Prentice-Hall.

150.   Greenblatt, E., Kirk, M. A., & Lehman, E. V. (2009). Restore yourself: the antidote for professional exhaustion. Execu-Care Books.

151.   Everly, G. S., Jr. Sherman, M. F., Stapleton, A., Barrett, D. J., Hiremath, G. S., & Links, J. M. (2006). Workplace crisis interventions: A systematic review of effect sizes. *Journal of Workplace Behavioral Health, 21*, 153-170.

152.   Fernandez, R. (2016). Five ways to boost your resilience at work. Harvard Business Review. Available on-line at: https://hbr.org/2016/06/627-building-resilience-ic-5-ways-to-build-your-personal-resilience-at-work

Chapter 21: The End of Shame

153.   Hermann, J. (1992). *Trauma and recovery: The aftermath of violence—from domestic abuse to political terror.* New York City, NY: BasicBooks

154.   Berkowitz, S., Stover, C., Marans, S. (2011). The child and family traumatic stress intervention: Secondary prevention for at risk youth of developing PTSD. *Journal of Child Psychology & Psychiatry*, 52(6); 676-685.

155.   Potter-Efron, P. S., & Potter-Efron, R. T. (1999). The secret message of shame: Pathways to hope and healing. Oakland, CA: New Harbinger Publications.

156.   Pivetti, M., Camodeca, M., & Rapino, M. (2016). Shame, guilt, and anger: Their cognitive, physiological, and behavioral correlates. *Current Psychology, 4*, 690-699.

157.   Launer, J. (2005). Anna O and the 'talking cure.' *QJM: An international Journal of medicine, 98*, 465-466.

158.   Brown, B. (2012). *Daring greatly: How the courage to be vulnerable transforms the way we live, love, parent, and lead.* New York City, NY: Avery.

159.   Cheavens, J. S., Cukrowicz, K. C., Hansen, R., & Mitchell, S. M. (2015). Incorporating resilience factors into the interpersonal theory of suicide: The role of hope and self-forgiveness in an older adult sample. *Journal of Clinical Psychology, 72*, 58-69.

Printed in the USA
CPSIA information can be obtained
at www.ICGtesting.com
JSHW082228140824
68134JS00017B/790